Rhinoplasty: Contemporary Innovations

Editor

RICHARD E. DAVIS

FACIAL PLASTIC SURGERY CLINICS OF NORTH AMERICA

www.facialplastic.theclinics.com

Consulting Editor
J. REGAN THOMAS

February 2015 • Volume 23 • Number 1

ELSEVIER

1600 John F. Kennedy Boulevard • Suite 1800 • Philadelphia, Pennsylvania, 19103-2899

http://www.theclinics.com

FACIAL PLASTIC SURGERY CLINICS OF NORTH AMERICA Volume 23, Number 1
February 2015 ISSN 1064-7406, ISBN-13: 978-0-323-35438-7

Editor: Joanne Husovski
Developmental Editor: Susan Showalter

Facial Plastic Surgery Clinics of North America (ISSN 1064-7406) is published quarterly by Elsevier Inc., 360 Park Avenue South, New York, NY 10010-1710. Months of issue are February, May, August, and November. Business and Editorial Offices: 1600 John F. Kennedy Blvd., Suite 1800, Philadelphia, PA 19103-2899. Periodicals postage paid at New York, NY, and additional mailing offices. Subscription prices are $390.00 per year (US individuals), $525.00 per year (US institutions), $445.00 per year (Canadian individuals), $653.00 per year (Canadian institutions), $535.00 per year (foreign individuals), $653.00 per year (foreign institutions), $185.00 per year (US students), and $255.00 per year (foreign students). Foreign air speed delivery is included in all *Clinics* subscription prices. All prices are subject to change without notice. POSTMASTER: Send address changes to *Facial Plastic Surgery Clinics*, Elsevier Health Sciences Division, Subscription Customer Service, 3251 Riverport Lane, Maryland Heights, MO 63043. **Customer service: 1-800-654-2452 (US and Canada); 1-314-447-8871 (outside US and Canada); Fax: 314-447-8029; E-mail:journalscustomerservice-usa@elsevier.com (for print support); journalsonline support-usa@elsevier.com (for online support).**

Reprints. For copies of 100 or more of articles in this publication, please contact the Commercial Reprints Department, Elsevier Inc., 360 Park Avenue South, New York, NY 10010-1710. Tel.: 212-633-3874; Fax: 212-633-3820; E-mail: reprints@elsevier.com.

Facial Plastic Surgery Clinics of North America is covered in *MEDLINE/PubMed* (*Index Medicus*).

Contributors

CONSULTING EDITOR

J. REGAN THOMAS, MD
Mansueto Professor and Chairman,
Department of Otolaryngology–Head and Neck
Surgery, University of Illinois at Chicago,
Chicago, Illinois

EDITOR

RICHARD E. DAVIS, MD, FACS
Director, The Center for Facial Restoration,
Miramar, Florida; Voluntary Professor, Division
of Facial Plastic Surgery, Department of
Otolaryngology–Head and Neck Surgery,
University of Miami Miller School of Medicine,
Miami, Florida

AUTHORS

PETER A. ADAMSON, MD, FACS, FRCSC
Professor and Head, Division of Facial Plastic
and Reconstructive Surgery, Department of
Otolaryngology–Head and Neck Surgery,
University of Toronto; Adamson Associates
Cosmetic Facial Surgery, Toronto, Ontario,
Canada

SCOTT A. ASHER, MD
Division of Facial Plastic and Reconstructive
Surgery, Department of Otolaryngology–Head
& Neck Surgery, University of Illinois at
Chicago, Chicago, Illinois

JAY CALVERT, MD
Assistant Clinical Professor, Division of Plastic
and Reconstructive Surgery, University of
Southern California, Beverly Hills, California

RICHARD E. DAVIS, MD, FACS
Director, The Center for Facial Restoration,
Miramar, Florida; Voluntary Professor, Division
of Facial Plastic Surgery, Department of

Otolaryngology–Head and Neck Surgery,
University of Miami Miller School of Medicine,
Miami, Florida

WOLFGANG GUBISCH, MD, PhD
Ärztlicher Direktor, Klinik für
Plast.Gesichtschirurgie, Marienhospital,
Stuttgart, Germany

BAHMAN GUYURON, MD
Kiehn-DesPrez Professor and Chair,
Department of Plastic Surgery, University
Hospitals Case Medical Center, Cleveland,
Ohio

KRISTOPHER KATIRA, MD
Resident, Department of Plastic Surgery,
University Hospitals Case Medical Center,
Cleveland, Ohio

MILOS KOVACEVIC, MD
HNO-Praxis am Hanse-Viertel, Hamburg,
Germany

EDWIN KWON, MD
Division of Plastic and Reconstructive Surgery,
University of Southern California, Beverly Hills,
California

NOAH BENJAMIN SANDS, MD, FRCSC
Clinical Fellow, Division of Facial Plastic
and Reconstructive Surgery,
Department of Otolaryngology–Head
and Neck Surgery, University of
Toronto; Adamson Associates Cosmetic
Facial Surgery, Toronto, Ontario, Canada

DEAN M. TORIUMI, MD
Division of Facial Plastic and
Reconstructive Surgery, Department of
Otolaryngology–Head & Neck Surgery,
University of Illinois at Chicago, Chicago,
Illinois

JOCHEN WURM, MD
Department of Otolaryngology–Head and Neck
Surgery, University Medical Center Erlangen,
Erlangen, Germany

Contents

Nasal hump excision is common during septorhinoplasty. Without appropriate restoration of the middle nasal vault, cosmetic and functional problems may ensue. Recently, spreader flaps have become an established alternative to traditional spreader grafts. Typical indications include primary rhinoplasty patients with hump noses, hump/tension noses, and moderately hooked or crooked noses. When suitable patients are selected, spreader flaps and their modifications represent a reliable alternative to the standard spreader graft, and when all of the necessary prerequisites are met, this technique obviates the need for additional cartilage grafting in most cases.

A septal deformity with severe deviation of the septal L strut is seen in nearly every crooked or scoliotic nose. Unless the underlying septal deformity is properly diagnosed and treated, the nasal axis cannot be completely straightened. In addition, because standard septoplasty techniques often fail to adequately address severe L-strut deformities, extracorporeal septoplasty is often a prerequisite for straightening the crooked nose. This article presents a detailed explanation of the extracorporeal technique, as well as representative long-term clinical results showing the efficacy and durability of extracorporeal septoplasty. Extracorporeal septoplasty a safe and reliable method for straightening the severely deviated nose.

Refinement of the wide, ptotic, under protected tip is one of the most difficult challenges in cosmetic nasal surgery yet also among the most common. Although excisional techniques can produce reductions in lobular width, long-term contour alterations are unpredictable and subject to stigmatic tip deformity. Preservation of natural tip support is a fundamental requirement of a successful rhinoplasty. The traditional lateral crural steal is a useful technique for tip refinement, but, when combined with a sturdy septal extension graft, the modified lateral crural steal (lateral crural tensioning) becomes a more potent and versatile rhinoplasty technique that can improve tip contour without jeopardizing function or structural stability.

After completion of this article, the reader should be able to describe the indications for lateral crural repositioning, understand the key steps to performing the procedure, and be able to manage the complications associated with this treatment strategy.

Diced cartilage with deep temporalis fascia (DC-F) graft has become a popular technique for reconstruction of the nasal dorsum. Cartilage can be obtained from the septum, ear, or costal cartilage when employing the DC-F technique. The complications seen with DC-F grafts tend to occur early in the surgeon's implementation of this technique. Management of the complications varies depending on the severity of the problem. This article gives an overview of both the technique and the complications commonly encountered.

 Videos of the tongue-and-groove technique accompany this article

The short nose deformity is a complex entity with diverse causes and variable characteristics. This article divides shortening into anterior and pan-nose shortening as well as mild, moderate, or severe. Mild anterior shortening can be corrected with shield grafting, whereas moderate to severe shortening can be corrected using septal extension grafts, composite grafts, or the tongue-and-groove technique. Ancillary technical considerations are reviewed. General principles of patient assessment and rhinoplasty execution are discussed. Surgical cases are presented, and pertinent aspects of preoperative planning, surgical technique, and perioperative care are discussed.

Vertical arch division is a mainstay of tip surgery, and its applications are expanding. It allows deprojection of the overprojected tip, and modifies rotation, length, and lobule definition. These parameters can be altered in a controlled, predictable fashion when the alar cartilage is preserved and overlapped, maintaining its strength. Cartilage overlay techniques aim to preserve normal anatomy and establish support for the nasal framework. We discuss the uses of vertical arch division when applied to the M-arch model, an expansion of the nasal tip tripod concept, which provides for a utilitarian approach to surgical techniques for the nasal tip.

FACIAL PLASTIC SURGERY CLINICS OF NORTH AMERICA

RELATED INTEREST

Clinics in Plastic Surgery, Volume 37, Issue 4, April 2010
Nasal and Facial Analysis
CR Woodard and SS Park, *Authors*
Ronald P. Gruber and David Stepnick, *Editors*

NOW AVAILABLE FOR YOUR iPhone and iPad

Preface
Rhinoplasty: Contemporary Innovations

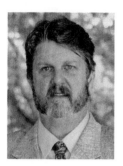

Richard E. Davis, MD, FACS
Editor

The human nose has a pivotal role in facial beauty. While an attractive and well-proportioned nose can enhance facial beauty by drawing attention to the eyes, a misshapen nose becomes obtrusive and diverts attention to the flawed nasal contour. Although a well-executed rhinoplasty has the potential to restore facial harmony, the unfavorable outcome can have an equally devastating impact on self-assurance, self-confidence, and self-esteem.

Given the emotional impact of rhinoplasty, coupled with the anatomic intricacy and functional importance of the nose, it's no surprise that rhinoplasty is now widely regarded as among the most difficult and enigmatic of all cosmetic surgeries. Yet despite the inherent challenges, the allure of enhanced facial beauty has propelled cosmetic nasal surgery to a new level of global popularity. Commensurate with this growth is an unprecedented surge in technical innovation and surgical efficacy. In fact, the last three decades probably account for more technical innovation than all other decades combined. As a consequence, the master nasal surgeon can now deliver favorable and longer-lasting results with greater consistency than at any other time in human history.

In this issue of *Facial Plastic Surgery Clinics of North America*, several of the world's preeminent

nasal surgeons share many of the innovations and insights that have helped to propel rhinoplasty to a new era of sophistication. I wish to personally thank the authors for their selfless generosity of thought and for their well-written technical descriptions. I'm confident that our readership will benefit from this issue of *Facial Plastic Surgery Clinics of North America*, and I trust you will enjoy reading these articles as much or more than I have. Indeed, the seeds of future innovation may well germinate from the concepts that follow.

Richard E. Davis, MD, FACS
Director, The Center for Facial Restoration
1951 Southwest 172nd Avenue, Suite 205
Miramar, FL 33029, USA

Voluntary Professor
Division of Facial Plastic Surgery
Department of Otolaryngology–Head & Neck Surgery
The University of Miami Miller School of Medicine
1120 Northwest 14th Street, 5th floor
Miami, FL 33136, USA

E-mail address:
drd@davisrhinoplasty.com

Facial Plast Surg Clin N Am 23 (2015) ix
http://dx.doi.org/10.1016/j.fsc.2014.10.001
1064-7406/15/$ – see front matter

Spreader Flaps for Middle Vault Contour and Stabilization

Milos Kovacevic, MD[a],[*],[1], Jochen Wurm, MD[b],[1]

KEYWORDS

- Spreader flap techniques • Spreader flaps • Spreader grafts • Inverted V deformity • Middle vault
- Internal nasal valve

KEY POINTS

- Reconstruction of the middle nasal vault after nasal hump removal is almost always necessary to prevent postoperative functional and cosmetic imperfections including the inverted V deformity.
- Spreader grafts are the gold standard for restoring the stability and contour of the middle vault after hump reduction; recently, spreader flaps have become reliable treatment alternative in select cases.
- Improvements and modifications of the basic spreader flap technique allow precise adjustments to middle vault contour to further expand the utility of spread flap reconstruction; however, appropriate patient selection is crucial to a satisfactory surgical outcome.

INTRODUCTION AND TREATMENT GOALS

A considerable number of patients who express the desire for cosmetic rhinoplasty require contouring and subsequent stabilization of the middle nasal vault. Some of these patients may present with an overly narrow humped middle vault and a (natural) visible delineation between the nasal bones and the upper lateral cartilages (ULC). Endonasal examination in these patients often reveals pinching of the internal nasal valve with an accompanying reduction in valve patency and premature collapse of the ULCs upon inspiration. This phenomenon is particularly common in patients who present with a high, peaked nasal dorsum, as seen in the so-called tension nose deformity. However, patients with short nasal bones, long and weak ULCs, and thin nasal skin are also at increased risk for middle vault distortion and collapse after nasal hump reduction. In fact,

surgical detachment of the ULC from the dorsal septum can incite pinching, malposition, and/or concave collapse of the ULC in virtually any nose, and when predisposing factors are not properly recognized and treated, unsightly cosmetic aftereffects of nasal surgery frequently occur. Typically, this manifests as inward collapse of the lateral nasal sidewalls (often accompanied by a slight middle vault saddle deformity) and symptomatic nasal airway obstruction. When the middle vault narrowing is severe in comparison to upper vault width, a stigmatic upside-down V-shaped shadow becomes visible at the bony–cartilaginous junction, an unsightly contour abnormality known as the "inverted V" deformity. In addition to the V-shaped shadow, the dorsal aesthetic lines are often disrupted or "washed out," particularly after over-resection of the dorsal hump.

The importance of maintaining a functional internal nasal valve and reconstructing the middle

[a] HNO-Praxis am Hanse-Viertel, Gerhofstrasse 2, Hamburg 20354, Germany; [b] Department of Otolaryngology, Head and Neck Surgery, University Medical Center Erlangen, Waldstrasse 1, Erlangen 91054, Germany
[1] Both authors contributed equally to this work.
* Corresponding author.
E-mail address: info@dr-kovacevic.de

Facial Plast Surg Clin N Am 23 (2015) 1–9
http://dx.doi.org/10.1016/j.fsc.2014.09.001

nasal vault immediately after hump reduction is now widely recognized among rhinoplasty experts.[1–9] The groundwork was laid by Sheen,[1] who first advocated spreader grafts for middle vault stabilization and contour enhancement. Today, spreader grafts have become the gold standard for preserving or restoring contour and structural integrity of the middle vault. However, the more recent advent of spreader flaps has added a second option for middle vault reconstruction after hump reduction in select patients. Instead of trimming the ULCs to match the newly established dorsal profile, the excess vertical height is used to create bilateral inwardly folded cartilage flaps that are sutured to the upper margin of the dorsal septum to strengthen and stabilize the surgically weakened middle vault. In principle, the in-folded ULCs behave similar to traditional spreader grafts by maintaining width at the apex of the nasal valve and thereby increasing the threshold for inspiratory nasal valve collapse. This benefit is derived almost entirely by the springlike effect of the partially folded ULCs, which mimic the natural anatomic configuration of a well-functioning ULC–septal junction. However, only patients with adequate ULC length and reasonably firm cartilage are satisfactory candidates for spreader flap fabrication.

Oneal and Berkowitz[10] first described the use of in-folded ULC flaps in 1998 and coined the term "spreader flaps." Later, further modifications were made, especially by Rohrich and colleagues, Byrd and colleagues,[11] Gruber and colleagues,[12,13] Ozmen and colleagues,[14] and Neu.[15] However, in our opinion, these modifications failed to fully optimize nasal valve function and airway patency. Furthermore, the modifications offered only limited opportunities for customization of the middle valve width according to the individual functional and cosmetic goals. The modifications we describe herein are further refinements of the spreader flap technique and serve to address these shortcomings.

PREOPERATIVE PLANNING AND PREPARATION

Preoperative findings and planned surgical objectives are discussed in detail with the patient, and objectives vary according to individual patient preferences. Patients are also fully informed about the risks and benefits of the planned procedure. Morphing software may be of value in this context, but the patient must be told that the images generated from such software are only approximations and by no means a guarantee of a particular postoperative result. Patients are also advised not take

any nonsteroidal anti-inflammatory drugs or anticoagulants for 10 to 14 days before surgery.

Immediate preoperative preparation includes cutting the nasal vibrisse and disinfecting the nasal vestibule. All incision and osteotomy lines are infiltrated with an injection solution containing 2% lidocaine and adrenaline 1:200,000 to minimize intraoperative bleeding.

SURGICAL TECHNIQUE
Basic Spreader Flaps

For surgical exposure, we routinely use the external rhinoplasty approach. This begins with degloving the entire skeletal framework in a sub-superficial musculoaponeurotic system (SMAS) dissection plane via a transcolumellar incision. Dissections should be carried out in a supraperichondrial and subperiosteal planes, respectively. Starting from the anterior septal angle, bilateral submucosal tunnels are then elevated on the undersurface of the ULC–septal cartilage junction and extended cranially beneath the bony vault. A "component" cartilaginous hump reduction is then begun by sharply dividing the ULC from the dorsal septum while preserving the underlying mucosa. In this manner, the overprojected ULC are not trimmed and can be used for spreader flap creation. Next, sharp reduction of the cartilaginous dorsal septum is performed to establish the new middle vault profile line. After resecting the cartilaginous septal hump, fibrous attachments of the ULC to the undersurface of the nasal bones are released in the midline using blunt dissection over an approximately 0.5-cm wide strip on both sides. Because the ULC release is confined to the area of planned bony hump resection, the detached cephalic ends of the ULC (which may extend as far as 10–12 mm beneath the rhinion) are protected during hump reduction, whereas the more lateral bony attachments of the ULC to the nasal bones remain intact. By preserving the uppermost extensions of the ULC, minor postoperative contour irregularities of the open roof can sometimes be prevented. After separation of the ULC and elevation of their perichondrium in 0.5- to 1-cm wide strip, both medial edges can be invaginated medially as turn-in flaps and temporarily positioned alongside the dorsal septum for suture fixation. Our method for flap fixation differs from previously described techniques. First, the distal rolled ends of the ULC are grasped and pulled caudally while they are sutured to the upper (caudal) border of dorsal septum (**Figs. 1** and **2**). As a rule, we find that 1 internal fixation suture is adequate for secure fixation. However, in cases of skeletal instability at the keystone area, a

1064-7406/... – see front matter © 201 Elsevier Inc. All rights reserved

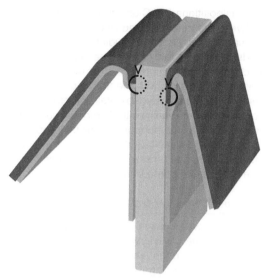

Fig. 1. Basic spreader flaps with internal anchoring suture.

second suture can be added cranially for additional stabilization. We prefer a 4-0 Polydioxanone suture for flap fixation. The knot is buried between the ULC and septum to prevent visible contour irregularities. Moreover, hiding the knot keeps a

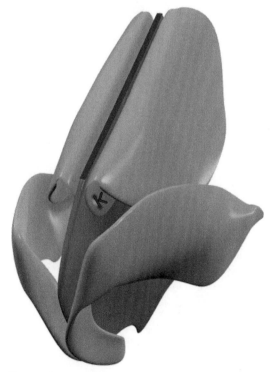

Fig. 2. Cross-section through the septum and the upper lateral cartilages after placement of basic spreader flaps.

possible foreign body reaction hidden beneath the skeletal framework. Care is taken to match spreader flap height to the existing height of the dorsal septum to create a smooth and straight dorsal profile. In virtually every case of spreader flap placement, in-folding and fixation of the ULC introduces modest laterally directed tension across the ULC. This beneficial tension tightens the ULC to minimize inward collapse and thereby helps to maintain and/or improve internal valve patency. Moreover, depending on the natural rigidity of the ULC, a springlike effect is often generated at the ULC fold that further contributes to valve patency and stabilization against sidewall collapse. In this way, spreader flaps can be used to reconstruct the contours and the functional stability of the middle vault after hump reduction. However, modifications of the basic technique can also be used for further contour refinements of the middle vault according to individual patient requirements.

Flaring-Type Spreader Flaps

Reconstruction of the middle nasal vault with basic spreader flaps may not always achieve the desired width and contour in some patients. In noses with an overprojected and ultranarrow dorsum, commonly seen in the tension nose deformity, additional widening of the middle nasal vault is often indicated for satisfactory airway function. Conversely, ultrawide or asymmetric noses may require additional narrowing to achieve satisfactory cosmetic results.

Our first modification of the basic technique was the "flaring"-type spreader flap. This modified spreader flap uses a horizontal mattress suture placed over top of the middle vault to suspend and flare the ULC as previously described by Park[16] (Fig. 3). However, we use horizontal mattress sutures instead of a vertical mattress suture to allow a more variable cartilage surface to be grasped and expanded. Tightening the flaring suture produces an incremental increase in the amount of lateral displacement of the ULC, thereby widening the middle vault and increasing valve patency. By adjusting final suture tension, middle vault width and valve patency can be fine tuned to the desired contour. Placement of the flaring suture is performed only after initial fixation of the basic spreader flap. The suture is first passed through the ULC in a caudal–cranial direction approximately 1 mm below the apex of the cartilage fold. Next, the suture is passed through the contralateral ULC in the equivalent position, but in the opposite direction. A large "purchase" is taken with each pass to prevent the suture

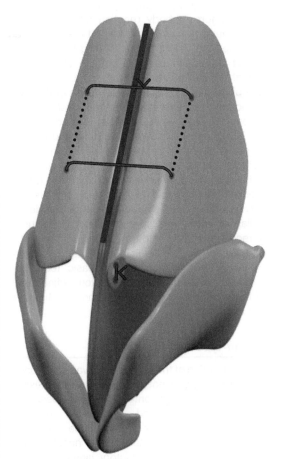

Fig. 3. Bilateral flaring-type spreader flaps.

the malpositioned ULC and the opposite ULC, or between the malpositioned ULC and the adjacent dorsal septum. Short, longitudinal incisions at both ends of the ULC fold can also be performed when a canoe-shaped contour of the middle vault is desired (**Fig. 4**). As with the flaring suture, suture tension can be adjusted to obtain incremental narrowing of middle vault width. And because the flaring suture and the support suture have opposite effect on middle vault width, variations in the number, position, and tension of these sutures can be used to custom contour the middle vault.

Postage-Stamp Spreader Flaps

In patients with unusually strong ULC, especially when combined with kinking, fracture lines, or protrusions, it is often impossible to achieve an aesthetically pleasing middle vault contour using the aforementioned spreader flap modifications. However, it is possible to decrease ULC rigidity with focal punctate stab incisions along the ULC fold to further enhance contour control (**Fig. 5**).

from tearing through the ULC. For this maneuver, 4-0 Polydioxanone is also recommended. Variations in suture placement and suture tension can be used to vary the dorsal lines of the middle vault, and by adding additional sutures at various points along the ULC, sidewall contour can be controlled with precision.

Support-Type Spreader Flaps

Our previous experience with the basic spreader flap technique confirmed its utility in the restoration of middle nasal vault contour.[9] However, in some patients, particularly those with rigid cartilage, the basic spreader flap may have a tendency toward excessive dorsal width. Conversely, there may also be preexisting asymmetries or deformities of the ULC that also require additional treatment. Hence, we have implemented a second modification that permits tailored reductions in middle vault width to further enhance contour control.

In areas where the middle vault is overly wide or where the cartilage vaulting is asymmetric, a (trans-septal) mattress suture is passed between

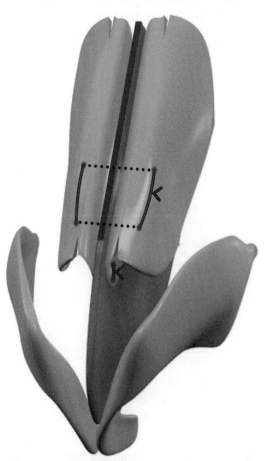

Fig. 4. Bilateral support-type spreader flaps with external mattress suture.

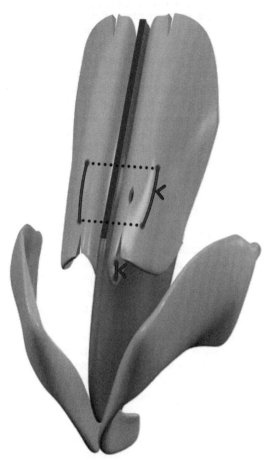

Fig. 5. Interrupted-type spreader flaps.

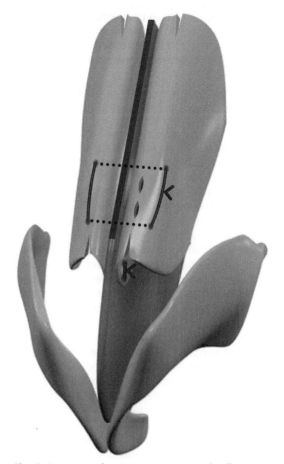

Fig. 6. Interrupted postage stamp spreader flaps.

Care must be taken to avoid complete division of the ULC because excessive destabilization may result in pinching and airway impingement. The focally weakened ULC can then be modified using one of the aforementioned suture techniques to restore ULC contour. We recommend single or multiple punctate stab incisions depending on the extent of the pathologic findings. Because more than 1 stab incision is often necessary, we have chosen to name this technique the "postage stamp spreader flap" (**Fig. 6**).

PATIENT SELECTION

The indications for using spreader flaps include previously unoperated noses with a prominent dorsal hump, tension nose deformity, or a mild to moderate crooked nose with a dorsal hump. In all cases, there must be sufficient vertical excess of the ULC to allow for sufficient in-folding while still maintaining adequate projection to establish the newly created profile line. This requirement is usually only met in patients with sizable rhinion humps. Spreader flaps are seldom possible after

previous dorsal hump resection or in saddle nose deformities.

In markedly crooked noses, deviation of the dorsal septum may persist despite septoplasty and nasal osteotomies. In these patients, the spreader flap techniques described may not fully eliminate the residual deformity or provide adequate splinting support owing to a lack of longitudinal rigidity. In such cases, splinting of the dorsal septum with traditional spreader grafts is usually required. Similarly, patients with pronounced facial asymmetry and unilateral shortening of the ULC are also poor candidates for spreader flap reconstruction. In these instances, unilateral augmentation grafting is often required to restore skeletal symmetry.

In our experience, not all patients with a prominent dorsal hump are favorable candidates for spreader flap reconstruction owing to thin, friable, and weak ULC. This is most commonly seen in pronounced tension nose deformities. Even though the excess vertical cartilage can be easily in-folded to create spreader flaps, the cartilage is too frail to withstand the rigors of postoperative scarring and soft tissue contracture. Irregularities in the contour of the middle nasal vault may then occur. Hence, robust spreader grafts should therefore be considered in these cases.

ADVANTAGES AND DISADVANTAGES OF SPREADER FLAP TECHNIQUES

Our technique of basic spreader flaps with internal fixation sutures presented herein provides a foundation for reliable reconstruction of the middle nasal vault. In contrast with the standard spreader flap techniques, the ULC are not weakened by extensive incisions or score marks. Thus, the natural cartilage tension is maintained, thereby optimizing stability of the middle vault. Moreover, middle vault contour can be restored without visibly sharp edges, often seen in spreader flaps secured with tight external mattress sutures, particularly in thin-skinned noses. The technique presented herein avoids this problem by creating a rounded infold, which mimics the configuration and vaulting of the natural ULC–septal junction. And unlike the standard spreader flap techniques, which have only limited capacity to control middle vault contour, the flaring, supporting, and interrupted techniques presented offer additional options for unilateral or bilateral fine tuning of the middle vault contour. Because spreader flaps obviate the need for donor cartilage, the demand for donor cartilage is reduced, and sparse septal donor tissue can be devoted to other needs. The risk of inadvertently weakening the septal L-strut is also reduced when septal graft tissue is no longer needed.

Despite the utility of spreader flap reconstruction in select patients, spreader graft reconstruction remains an indispensable treatment option for a large percentage of rhinoplasty patients, particularly revision rhinoplasty patients. Perhaps the most common indication for spreader grafting is a nose that has already undergone dorsal hump excision. In such cases, the excess vertical height of ULC is no longer available to fashion spreader flaps and other means of middle vault stabilization are required. Moreover, even if hump reduction was not performed as part of the primary rhinoplasty, scarring of the middle vault may sometimes make sufficient mobilization of the ULC difficult or impossible. Perhaps the most obvious indication for spreader graft reconstruction is the patient presenting with a conspicuous inverted V deformity in which middle vault reconstruction was inadequate or neglected entirely. In these cases, very strong spreader grafts are needed to stabilize and contour the middle vault, and even when there is still adequate ULC available, spreader flaps seldom meet the anatomic requirements for middle vault reconstruction. Finally, our experience has also shown that a subgroup of primary rhinoplasty patients with dorsal overprojection may not make good candidates for spreader flap reconstruction. These patients include those with pronounced tension nose deformities, markedly crooked noses, saddle nose deformities, and those with significant mid face asymmetry. In this patient population, the need for spreader grafts (and the additional donor cartilage) should be included as part of the initial surgical plan.

POSSIBLE COMPLICATIONS AND THEIR MANAGEMENT

In rhinoplasty, achieving a stable, symmetric, and attractive middle vault contour after hump reduction is difficult, and satisfactory long-term results are difficult to achieve with any surgical technique. Typically, when middle vault support is inadequate, the ULC collapse medially, producing an inverted V deformity. However, in more than 600 spreader flaps cases using the techniques described herein, we have yet to observe a single case of inverted V deformity.[17] Mild asymmetries in sidewall slope or circumscribed depression of the dorsum at the bony–cartilaginous junction have occurred in only 3% of cases.[17] However, we now use shaved cartilage paste, which is obtained by harvesting paper-thin slices of septal cartilage, to camouflage these contour irregularities. Additionally, we observed a slight tendency for excessive middle vault width after the basic or flaring spreader flap technique, for a revision rate of 0.5%.[16] However, these cases were successfully treated by the addition of a support-type external mattress suture to achieve the desired middle vault width.

We also observed widening of the middle vault in 4% of cases treated with support or interrupted-type spreader flaps.[17] This paradoxical outcome was initially difficult to explain until a detailed case review revealed that the problem was limited almost exclusively to patients with a slight bony cartilaginous hump. In these patients, very little excess ULC was available for spreader flap formation, and even with subperichondrial release of the ULC, the recruitment of ULC was insufficient to prevent excessive lateral tension on the newly fashioned spreader flaps. Because the nasal bones were fully mobilized after osteotomies, the laterally based tension, combined with postoperative swelling, led to gradual splaying and widening of the nasal dorsum. The splaying was also more pronounced in noses where the ULC attachments to the nasal bones extended more than 4 mm above the caudal bony margin.

Unfortunately, the availability of excess ULC for spreader graft formation (after resection of a small nasal hump) cannot be determined until the cartilage is fully mobilized. Although adequate recruitment is possible in some noses, spreader flaps should not be used when the fixation suture results in excessive lateral tension, and preoperative planning should include a contingency for spreader graft placement in all noses with small dorsal humps.

POSTPROCEDURAL CARE

Upon completion, the transcolumellar and marginal incisions are closed and bilateral septal splints are inserted for 1 week. Nasal packing is usually unnecessary, but a thermoplastic splint is applied to the nasal dorsum. Prophylactic antibiotics are administered as a single dose during surgery. Decongestant nasal drops are also used 3 times per day for 1 week. A specially prepared emulsion containing menthol and lanolin is applied in the nasal cavity in the same fashion. Bandage removal is performed after 7 days, and as a rule, no further treatment measures are required.

CASE STUDIES
Case One

A young white woman presented for primary rhinoplasty. Examination revealed a long nose with a prominent bony cartilaginous hump and a ptotic nasal tip (**Fig. 7**A, B). Endonasal examination revealed deviation of the nasal septum.

Using an external rhinoplasty approach, we first resected the cartilaginous and bony humps while preserving both ULC. After septoplasty, medial (parasagittal), transverse, and lateral osteotomies

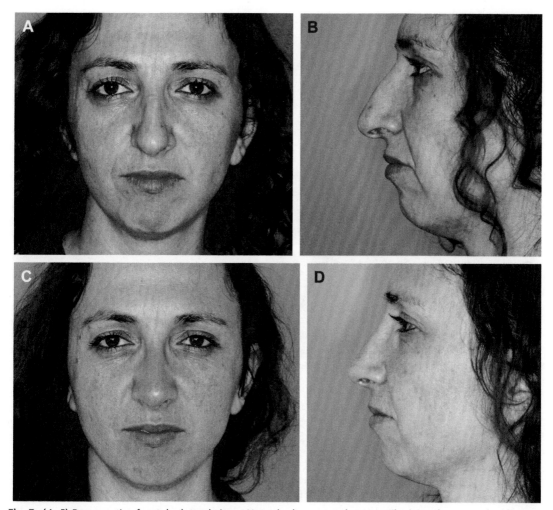

Fig. 7. (*A, B*) Preoperative frontal a lateral views. Note the long nose, bony-cartilaginous hump, and wide ptotic nasal tip. (*C, D*) Postoperative frontal and lateral views at 21 months. Note the strong and smooth middle vault with aesthetically pleasing dorsal aesthetic lines and no evidence of inverted V deformity.

were then used to close the open roof deformity. Reconstruction of the middle vault was achieved using bilateral interrupted spreader flaps. Tip refinement was accomplished using transposition of both lateral crura (including trimming of cartilage from the inferior margin) combined with a tongue-in-groove setback. Shaved cartilage paste was then used to camouflage minor irregularities of the dorsum.

The postoperative result at 21 months reveals a strong middle vault with smooth, aesthetically pleasing dorsal aesthetic lines and no signs of inverted V deformity (see **Fig. 7**C, D).

Case Two

A young white woman presented for primary rhinoplasty. Examination revealed a C-shaped nose with a wide and asymmetric nasal dorsum and a broad, asymmetric, and overprojected nasal tip (**Fig. 8**A, B).

Using the open rhinoplasty approach, the dorsum was lowered with preservation of the excess ULC. The bony vault was then straightened and narrowed using medial (oblique) and lateral osteotomies, and bilateral support spreader grafts were used to reconstruct and stabilize the middle vault. Tip deprojection and refinement was achieved with transposition of the lower lateral cartilages including a turn-under flap of the inferior margin.

The postoperative result at 14 months reveals a straight and symmetric dorsum with appropriate middle vault width and valve patency and no sign of inverted V deformity (see **Fig. 8**C, D).

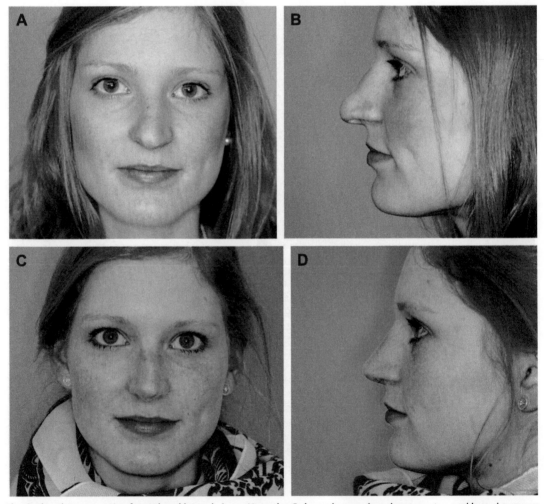

Fig. 8. (*A, B*) Preoperative frontal and lateral views. Note the C-shaped nose, dorsal asymmetry, and broad overprojected nasal tip. (*C, D*) Postoperative frontal a lateral views at 14 months. Note the straight dorsum, adequate middle vault width, and absence of inverted V deformity. The patient also had satisfactory internal nasal valve patency.

SUMMARY

Nasal hump excision is a very common procedure during septorhinoplasty. However, without appropriate restoration of the middle nasal vault, both cosmetic and functional problems may ensue. In recent years, spreader flaps have become an established alternative to traditional spreader grafts in the reconstruction of this important anatomic area. Typical indications for spreader flaps include primary rhinoplasty patients with hump noses, hump/tension noses, and moderately hooked or crooked noses. Basic, flaring, support, and interrupted-type spreader flaps can increase the available treatment options for fine tuning the middle nasal vault to meet individual cosmetic and functional requirements. When suitable patients are selected, spreader flaps and their modifications represent a reliable alternative to the standard spreader graft, and when all of the necessary prerequisites are met, this technique obviates the need for additional cartilage grafting in most cases.

REFERENCES

1. Sheen JH. Spreader graft: a method of reconstructing the roof of the middle nasal vault following rhinoplasty. Plast Reconstr Surg 1984; 73(2):230–9.
2. Rohrich RJ, Muzaffar AR, Janis JE. Component dorsal hump reduction: the importance of maintaining dorsal aesthetic lines in rhinoplasty. Plast Reconstr Surg 2004;114(5):1298–308.
3. Fischer H, Gubisch W. Nasal valves–importance and surgical procedures. Facial Plast Surg 2006;22(4): 266–80.
4. Ingels KJ, Orhan KS, van Heerbeek N. The effect of spreader grafts on nasal dorsal width in patients with nasal valve insufficiency. Arch Facial Plast Surg 2008;10(5):354–6.
5. Riedel F, Bran G. Cartilage grafts in functional and aesthetic rhinoplasty. HNO 2008;56(2):185–98.
6. Rohrich RJ, Hollier LH. Use of spreader grafts in the external approach to rhinoplasty. Clin Plast Surg 1996;23(2):255–62.
7. Sykes JM. Management of the middle nasal third in revision rhinoplasty. Facial Plast Surg 2008;24(3): 339–47.
8. Davis RE, Bublik M. Common technical causes of the failed rhinoplasty. Facial Plast Surg 2012;28(4): 380–9.
9. Toriumi DM. Subtotal septal reconstruction: an update. Facial Plast Surg 2013;29(6):492–501.
10. Oneal RM, Berkowitz RL. Upper lateral cartilage spreader flaps in rhinoplasty. Aesthet Surg J 1998; 18(5):370–1.
11. Byrd HS, Meade RA, Gonyon DL Jr. Using the autospreader flap in primary rhinoplasty. Plast Reconstr Surg 2007;119(6):1897–902.
12. Gruber RP, Park E, Newman J, et al. The spreader flap in primary rhinoplasty. Plast Reconstr Surg 2007;119(6):1903–10.
13. Gruber RP, Perkins SW. Humpectomy and spreader flaps. Clin Plast Surg 2010;37(2):285–91.
14. Ozmen S, Ayhan S, Findikcioglu K, et al. Upper lateral cartilage fold-in flap: a combined spreader and/or splay graft effect without cartilage grafts. Ann Plast Surg 2008;61(5):527–32.
15. Neu BR. Use of the upper lateral cartilage sagittal rotation flap in nasal dorsum reduction and augmentation. Plast Reconstr Surg 2009;123(3):1079–87.
16. Park SS. The flaring suture to augment the repair of the dysfunctional nasal valve. Plast Reconstr Surg 1998;101(4):1120–2.
17. Wurm J, Kovacevic M. A new classification of spreader flap techniques. Facial Plast Surg 2013; 29(6):506–14.

Treatment of the Scoliotic Nose with Extracorporeal Septoplasty

 CrossMark

Wolfgang Gubisch, MD, PhD

KEYWORDS

- Septal deformity • Septal correction • Septal reconstruction • Septoplasty • Nasal deformity
- Deviated nose • Breathing impairment

KEY POINTS

- Successful correction of the crooked nose requires a straight and sturdy L strut.
- Traditional septoplasty techniques are often ineffective at correcting deviation and deformities of the L strut.
- Contemporary rhinoplasty techniques made possible by the open rhinoplasty approach permit effective reconstruction of the deformed septal L strut.
- In severe cases, extracorporeal reconstruction in which the septal partition is removed from the nose, reconstructed, and then reimplanted, is necessary to achieve a strong, flat, and size-appropriate neoseptum and a straight nose.

INTRODUCTION

The idea of removing a severely deformed septum, reconstructing it on the table, and reimplanting the neoconstruct back into the nose was first published by King and Ashley[1] in 1951. The concept of extracorporeal septal reconstruction was then revisited in the early 1990s to treat stubborn deformities of the anterior septal L strut.[2–6] We have since refined the original technique to include en bloc removal of the bony-cartilaginous partition, creation of a flat and rigid L-strut replacement graft using autologous graft material (preferably salvaged from the septal partition), and secure fixation of the neoseptum to both the bony and cartilaginous skeletal framework. In the nearly 3 decades since we began performing extracorporeal septoplasty, much has changed with our technique. At present, we routinely perform extracorporeal septoplasty as part of a complete septorhinoplasty, including tip-plasty and/or dorsal hump reduction with full mobilization of the nasal bones. Although some surgeons regard extracorporeal reconstruction as unacceptable risk because of aggressive skeletal destabilization, particularly when extracorporeal septoplasty is performed in conjunction with complete nasal osteotomies, in our clinical experience, extracorporeal septal reconstruction performed as a stand-alone procedure or as part of a complete septorhinoplasty is a safe, effective, and reliable means for correcting severe L-strut deformities, and complications stemming from excessive destabilization have been rare. However, unlike our initial extracorporeal technique, we no longer use the closed rhinoplasty approach and now perform extracorporeal septoplasty exclusively through the external (open) rhinoplasty approach. The improved exposure associated with the open approach allows vastly improved surgical access, which in turn permits secure suture fixation of the neoseptum to the bony and cartilaginous skeletal framework. Although we previously sutured the neoseptum only to the upper lateral cartilages

Disclosure: The author receives royalties as a consultant of Medicon Company, Tuttlingen, Germany.
Klinik für Plast.Gesichtschirurgie, Marienhospital, Böheimstr.37, Stuttgart D-70199, Germany
E-mail address: wolfgang.gubisch@vinzenz.de

Facial Plast Surg Clin N Am 23 (2015) 11–22
http://dx.doi.org/10.1016/j.fsc.2014.09.002
1064-7406/15/$ – see front matter © 2015 Elsevier Inc. All rights reserved.

facialplastic.theclinics.com

(ULCs), we now also suture the neoseptum directly to the nasal bones (**Fig. 1**) and to the anterior nasal spine via small osseous drill holes (**Fig. 2**). Often we also drill a sagittal groove in the nasal spine for improved stabilization of the inferior caudal septum, and when necessary the bony nasal spine is transected at its base, relocated to the sagittal midline, and reattached with microplates and microscrews in order to ensure accurate midline positioning of the columellar pedestal (**Fig. 3**). Internal nasal valve patency is also enhanced using spreader grafts or spreader flaps in virtually every extracorporeal septoplasty, simultaneously enhancing both structural stability and nasal airway function.

Modification of the original extracorporeal septoplasty technique described herein has improved the efficacy of extracorporeal septoplasty and simultaneously reduced complications associated with treatment of the scoliotic nose. When performed correctly, the extracorporeal septoplasty, which is perhaps better termed extracorporeal septal reconstruction, is a reliable technique for straightening the twisted or deviated nose, and the modified technique has transformed the treatment of this previously challenging patient population.

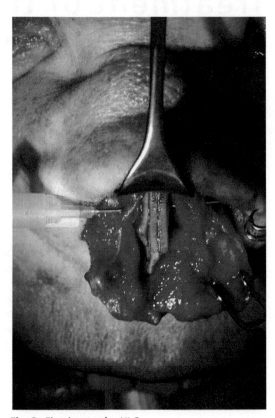

Fig. 2. Fixation to the ULC.

INDICATIONS

Although the septum is the central element of the nasal framework, its importance is often overlooked in nasal surgery. Even now, many otolaryngologists are erroneously taught that a septoplasty is a suitable operation for the beginner and requires only 20 to 30 minutes to complete. However, not all septal deformities are amenable to correction with straightforward septoplasty techniques. Although septal deformities that are

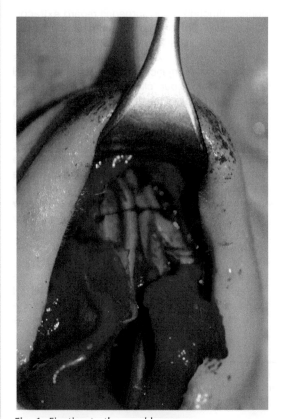

Fig. 1. Fixation to the nasal bones.

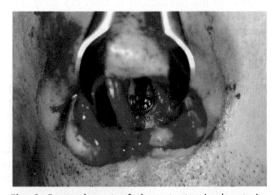

Fig. 3. Reattachment of the osteotomized anterior nasal spine with microplate and microscrews.

localized to the inferior/posterior aspect of the quadrangular septum can often be corrected with straightforward septoplasty techniques, these modest deformities cause only airway obstruction and do not produce deformities of the external nose. In contrast, complex septal deformities involving the outer septal L strut often produce both functional and cosmetic deformities, and these more severe septal deformities typically resist correction with traditional septoplasty techniques. Severe L-strut deformities are often impossible to eliminate with traditional septoplasty or rhinoplasty techniques. In contrast, not every septal deformity is responsible for the patient's complaint of airway dysfunction, and a complete nasal examination, coupled with diagnostic testing, is necessary to localize alternative sources of airway dysfunction such as nasal valve collapse or turbinate hypertrophy. In addition, although a perfectly straight septal partition is seldom required for adequate nasal airway function, a perfectly flat and midline L-strut partition is a prerequisite for a straight, symmetric, and properly aligned outer nose. The importance of a straight septal L strut is often underappreciated by cosmetic nasal surgeons, who are primarily concerned with the aesthetic outcome and who often fail to recognize the contribution of the outer nasal septum to the cosmetic result. As a result, the preoperative assessment must seek to identify deformities within the septal L strut in order to devise a comprehensive and effective treatment plan.

According to the classification system described by Guyuron,[7] septal deviations can be subdivided into 6 different types of anatomic deformity. C-shaped or S-shaped anterior-posterior septal deviations may lead to deformities of the dorsal L strut, whereas C-shaped or S-shaped cephalocaudal deviations can lead to deformities of the caudal (anterior) L strut. The remaining 2 classifications do not involve the L strut. Although some L-strut deformities can be treated effectively with traditional nonextracorporeal techniques, when properly executed the extracorporeal septal reconstruction can eliminate virtually any L-strut deformity and the extracorporeal technique remains the gold standard for severe anatomic derangements of the septal L strut.

SURGICAL TECHNIQUE
Dissection and en Bloc Removal of the Deformed Septum

In order to vasoconstrict the nasal mucosa, we prefer 2% ropivacaine, which is the only commercially available local anesthetic with intrinsic vasoconstrictive properties. For additional vasoconstriction the ropivacaine is mixed with epinephrine at a final concentration of 1:100,000. Following careful injection of the septal mucosa and the cutaneous incision lines, we obtain surgical access via the open (external) rhinoplasty approach. Because asymmetric scars are best avoided in the facial midline, we start with bilateral marginal incisions for dissecting the tip blindly, before we connect the marginal incisions with the transcolumellar incision, the upper membranous septum is dissected to expose the anterior septal angle, formed by the junction of the dorsal and caudal L struts. Once the anterior septal angle is identified, we elevate the mucoperichondrium with sharp-tipped scissors and begin blindly elevating tunnels along the dorsal septum at its junction with the ULCs. Once the septal/ULC junction has been denuded of mucosa, both ULCs are severed from the dorsal septum taking care not to injure the underlying nasal mucosa. A swivel-headed suction elevator is then used to extend the submucosal tunnels cranially beneath the nasal bones. In previously operated noses or in cases of severe anterior septal deformity, we have found that dissection is often easier when performed in an anterior-to-posterior direction using 2 parallel pairs of tunnels: one pair of tunnels along the dorsal septum and another pair just above the nasal floor. In the next step we consequently create separate inferior septal tunnels, starting at the piriform aperture, using a small periosteal elevator specifically designed for this purpose (**Fig. 4**). In addition, both tunnels are gradually joined in an anterior-to-posterior direction until the mucoperichondrial/mucoperiosteal flaps are completely elevated on both sides of the septal partition.

In most cases, before removing the septal partition we create parallel medial osteotomy cuts

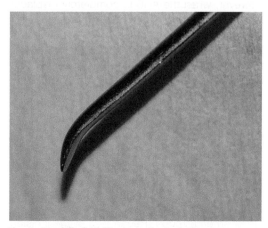

Fig. 4. Modified McKenty periosteal elevator.

using an electric drill fitted with a narrow Lindeman bur equipped with both side-cutting and end-cutting capacity (**Fig. 5**). In addition to creating perfect parasagittal osteotomy cuts for a straight and symmetric bony infracture, the Lindeman bur also removes small amounts of bone to produce a slender open-roof deformity in order to facilitate adequate narrowing of wide or stubborn nasal bones following both transverse and lateral osteotomies. In addition, the Lindeman bur is also used to make a 45° downward diagonal cut across the perpendicular ethmoid plate in order to reduce the risk of inadvertent cribriform disruption when fracturing the vertical ethmoid bone. Inferiorly, the maxillary crest and vomer are cut horizontally (beginning immediately posterior to the incisive foramen) using a 5-mm chisel. A posterior vertical fracture is then created by pressing firmly against the posterior bony septum with the 5-mm chisel. Care is taken to release all soft tissue attachments before attempting en bloc removal of the septal partition.

Analysis and Correction of a Malpositioned Anterior Nasal Spine

The next step is the assessment of the anterior nasal spine (ANS). In many patients with a severely deformed septum, and in all patients with a unilateral cleft nose, the ANS is displaced from the midline prohibiting fixation of the caudal septum in the sagittal midline. Our treatment algorithm depends on both the extent of bony displacement and the width of the ANS. If there is only minor displacement and the ANS is sufficiently wide (and at least partly in the midline), it can be narrowed on the protruding side using a cylindric cutting drill so that the residual bone rests in the midline. Transverse drill holes are then created in the residual ANS and suture fixation is used to secure the reimplanted caudal L strut in the midline. However, when the ANS is completely displaced

from the sagittal midline, we use the Lindeman bur to transect the ANS at its base, releasing the ANS from the premaxilla but leaving it pedicled anteriorly to the soft tissues. The ANS is then repositioned in the sagittal midline and reattached with an angled 4-hole microplate and two 3-mm to 5-mm microscrews (see **Fig. 3**). Because the ANS is no longer large enough to permit placement of transverse drill holes, the reimplanted caudal septum is usually sutured directly to the microplate for midline fixation.

Septal Reconstruction: Creation of a Neoseptum

The reconstruction of a straight neoseptum varies according to the septal deformity. In many cases, the caudal septum is severely deflected and must be excised. The remaining septum can usually be rotated by 90° such that the existing bony-cartilaginous (B-C) junction becomes the new dorsal septum. The desired length of the dorsal septum is predetermined using measurements from the native septum. Although straight, the B-C junction is usually thicker on one side, which necessitates either augmentation of the deficient side or thinning of the thickened side with a cylindrical bur. If the residual septum has a sufficiently large quadrangular cartilage, the septum can be cut approximately 5 mm below the B-C junction leaving a residual strip for use in augmentation of the deficient side or for use as a unilateral spreader graft, sometimes pedicled on perichondrium. As an alternative, spreader grafts can be fabricated from the resected portions of the deformed caudal septum or from surplus cartilage harvested away from the neo–L strut. However, when only crooked cartilage segments are available for spreader graft fabrication, the cylindrical drill can sometimes be used to eliminate thickened segments and produce a suitable spreader graft. Otherwise the deformed cartilage segments can be scored and splinted using perforated ethmoid bone grafts. Care must be taken to create as many drill holes as possible within the ethmoid bone so as to facilitate both suture fixation and optimal vascular and fibrous tissue ingrowth. When ethmoid bone is unavailable, bent segments of cartilage can be straightened using horizontal mattress sutures as described by Gruber and colleagues.[8] In addition, in the severely deformed septum, multiple small flat segments can be harvested and splinted with perforated ethmoid bone or polydioxanone (PDS) plate to create a mosaiclike neo–L strut.[9]

In the previously operated nose in which nearly all of the septal cartilage is absent but sufficient vomerine and/or ethmoid bone is available to

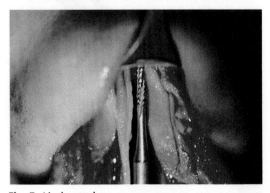

Fig. 5. Lindeman bur.

create an L strut of appropriate size, we thin the donor bone where necessary and create as many drill holes as possible without jeopardizing structural stability. In addition to making fixation easier, multiple drill holes promote better revascularization and stabilization by the ingrowth of fibrous tissue. They also permit transfixion sutures, which are sometimes added for additional structural stability. If no cartilage or bone is available to create a stable and flat L strut, the entire neoseptal construct must be created from either bilateral conchal grafts or from costal cartilage.

Creation of a Neoseptum Entirely from Conchal Cartilage

When sufficient nasal graft material is unavailable to permit construction of a strong and straight L-shaped neoseptum, both conchal donor sites can be used for septal reconstruction. The concha is harvested as a single en bloc specimen from each ear, and the convex side of each graft is sutured back to back with its counterpart using several longitudinal rows of running suture. To facilitate suture placement, a modified Aiach clamp is used to immobilize the grafts in a flat and symmetric orientation (**Fig. 6**). After suture fixation, the newly created sandwich graft remains flat and stabile, and the edges can be trimmed to create a smooth straight edge to form the L strut. When necessary, portions of the graft not contributing to the L strut can be excised and used for other purposes.

Straightening of the Deformed Bony Pyramid

Before reinserting the newly fabricated neoseptum, we prefer to mobilize and straighten the bony nasal pyramid. The medial osteotomies, which we perform as parallel sagittally oriented (parasagittal) cuts, are performed first in order to

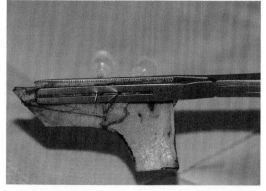

Fig. 6. Gubisch/Aiach clamp for graft immobilization during suturing.

control the width and alignment of the central bony complex. The bony nasal sidewalls are then aggressively mobilized using both transverse and lateral osteotomies, which are performed using the percutaneous technique. A sharpened 2-mm or 3-mm chisel is preferred for percutaneous osteotomies because it limits blunt-force energy transmission and reduces the likelihood of comminution, which is often seen with other methods. After making a single stab incision to access the entire osteotomy line, we use the chisel as a periosteal elevator to displace the overlying blood vessels and reduce the probability of bleeding. In most cases, the lateral osteotomy line begins low beneath the Webster triangle and remains low within the nasofacial groove until it terminates at the intercanthal line. We typically make no attempt to preserve the Webster triangle because we think that the functional implications are generally negligible, hence the designation of a low-to-low lateral osteotomy. In addition, we avoid the postage-stamp technique in which the perforations are separated by small strips of bone, and instead create a continuous uninterrupted lateral osteotomy cut fashioned from multiple connecting bony perforations. We then perform the transverse percutaneous osteotomy along the intercanthal line to fully mobilize the bony sidewall.

Implantation of the Neoseptum

After appropriate mobilization and positioning of the nasal bones, we then reimplant the neoseptum. Secure fixation of the neoseptum is a critical part of this process. Whenever the nasal bones can be exposed via retraction of the overlying skin envelope, albeit is possible to create drill holes in the nasal bones that allow suture fixation of the septal construct directly to the bony skeleton (see **Fig. 1**). Reimplantation begins with initial positioning of the septal construct, after which we use small needles to temporarily pin the construct to the ULC. Needles are sometimes passed percutaneously in order to best stabilize the construct. Once the complex is properly positioned, we create a transverse drill hole through the upper (caudal) border of the nasal bone above the keystone area. A 4-0 round needle is then passed transversely through the drill hole until it makes contact with the contralateral nasal bone, and this spot is marked for creation of the contralateral drill hole. After creating the second drill hole, the fixation suture is passed through the paired drill holes including the neoseptum, and then back through the adjacent ULC (or back through an additional pair of adjacent drill holes) and tied. This mattress fixation suture serves to bridge the keystone area and to secure the upper end of the neoseptum to the nasal bones. If the nasal bones are too short to permit access for drill hole placement, then we create osseous drill holes in a percutaneous fashion. The osseous drill holes are created by mounting a large-bore needle to the drill, penetrating the skin with the needle, and then creating drill holes through both nasal bones and the neoseptum using the large-bore needle. The needle is then left in position but disconnected from the drill and a 4-0 PDS suture is fed retrograde (subcutaneously) through the needle tip until it emerges from the needle hub. The needle is then removed and a small hook is passed subcutaneously to retrieve the suture end from beneath the skin flap so that it can be tied over the bony dorsum to stabilize the upper end of the neoseptum (Haack S, personal communication, 2013). Additional fixation of the construct to the ULCs is then performed taking care to keep the suture track below the upper edge of the neodorsum in case small reductions in septal height are necessary. The third and final point of fixation is to the ANS, which is first perforated with a Lindeman bur to create 1 or more transverse drill holes for osseous fixation. The desired dorsal height now depends on the length of the caudal L strut. Because we typically create a caudal segment that is longer than desired, we can reduce its length until the desired projection is achieved. Whenever possible we also create a shallow sagittally oriented groove in the ANS for stabilization of the caudal segment. Once the desired height is achieved with the caudal segment resting in the midline groove, suture fixation is performed with at least 3 passes using a 4-0 or 5-0 nonabsorbable suture. When ANS size permits, we also create more than 1 drill hole for additional stabilization. Passing the fixation suture through different points of the caudal segment and different holes within the ANS reduces the likelihood of unwanted rotation and/or displacement of the neoseptum. Hence, secure immobilization of the neoseptum is achieved through multipoint osseous suture fixation.

FINAL ADJUSTMENTS
Camouflage Techniques

After redraping the skin flap we palpate the dorsum to assess for irregularities. If irregularities are detected they can be smoothed with the cylindrical drill or camouflaged with allogenic fascia lata (Tutoplast, Tutogen) or finely diced cartilage (FDC) paste (Fig. 7). Because patients frequently refuse harvest of autologous fascia lata, and because autologous deep temporalis fascia is

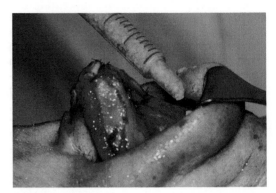
Fig. 7. FDC paste.

often too thin, our favorite method of dorsal camouflage is autologous FDC paste.[10] FDC is injected via the marginal incisions after the columellar incision is closed. We use a specifically developed tool for injection of FDC to avoid reelevation of the skin flap (Fig. 8).

Bandaging

For additional stabilization of the septal construct we place a running transseptal quilting suture of 4-0 PDS on a short Keith needle. This suture is followed by placement of bilateral silicone splints and foam packing impregnated with Otriven (xylometazoline hypochloride) and gentamicin antibiotic solution. The foam packing is removed on the second or third postoperative day, and a nasal cast fashioned from plaster of Paris and extending onto the forehead is secured with a gauze head wrap and maintained for 2 weeks to prevent widening of the nasal bones (Fig. 9).

ANCILLARY PROCEDURES
Treatment of Columellar Retraction

Correcting deformities of the anterior septum by resecting the caudal septum often results in columellar retraction unless the caudal septum is reconstructed primarily. In revision surgery, the

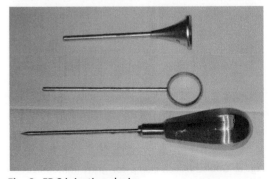
Fig. 8. FDC injection device.

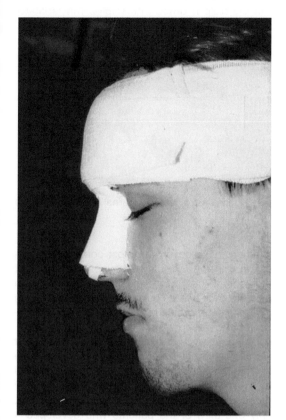

Fig. 9. Nasal cast fixed to the forehead with a circular bandage to reduce mimetic movement.

most effective means of reconstructing a retracted columella (characterized by inadequate columellar show and an overly acute nasolabial angle) is often a double-layered conchal graft placed directly in front of the anterior septal remnant to replace the missing caudal segment (**Figs. 10** and **11**). The graft is fabricated by harvesting the entire concha cymba (including the posterior perichondrium) and then dividing the cartilage along its longitudinal

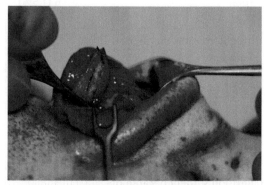

Fig. 10. Double-layered conchal graft in front of an overshortened anterior septum.

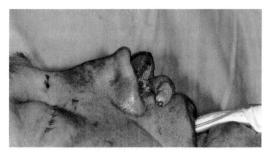

Fig. 11. Diced cartilage in fascia for premaxillary augmentation (DC-F)-graft.

centerline while keeping the perichondrium intact. Next, the graft is hinged on itself with the convex sides oriented back to back, and then sutured flat using several rows of running monofilament suture oriented parallel to the long axis. A modified Aiach clamp is also used to stabilize and flatten the bivalved segments during suture fixation. Once sutured, the flat and rigid bilaminar graft can be contoured to the desired size and outer contour. Care is taken to achieve a precise contour match between the back edge of the conchal graft and the leading edge of the caudal septum, and to contour the leading edge of the conchal graft to control the columellar profile.

When performing an extracorporeal septoplasty, columellar retraction can also be eliminated by extending the caudal septum forward to increase columellar projection. In this circumstance, the L strut is designed to have a longer dorsal component such that the caudal septum rests anterior to the ANS. In order to stabilize the base of the modified L strut in the midline, a groove is first cut into the face of the ANS to assist in transosseous suture fixation.

Augmentation of the Premaxilla with a Diced Cartilage in Fascia Graft

The most effective method for correcting severe columellar retraction and/or premaxillary hypoplasia with a hyper-acute nasolabial angle is augmentation with a premaxillary diced cartilage in fascia (DC-F) graft.[10] Although the DC-F graft was originally intended for use in augmentation of the collapsed or over-resected nasal dorsum, it is equally effective at correcting hypoplasia of the premaxilla (see **Fig. 11**). Cartilage for the premaxillary DC-F graft can be obtained from the rib cage, conchal bowl, or quadrangular septum, but we prefer to reserve the uniquely thin and flat septal cartilage for other purposes. Regardless of the cartilage source, it is essential to cut the donor cartilage into small cubes measuring 0.5 mm^3 or less using a sharp dermatome blade. To create the fascial sleeve, either autologous deep temporalis fascia or allogenic fascia lata (Tutoplast, Tutogen) is sewn around a tuberculin syringe. After suturing the distal end closed and filling the fascial sleeve with the diced ear and/or rib cartilage, the opposite end of the sleeve is also sutured shut. Before reimplantation of the neoseptum, a pocket is created over the premaxilla via the external rhinoplasty approach and the DC-F is inserted through the membranous septum into the premaxillary pocket. No fixation of the DC-F graft is required because the pocket size corresponds closely with the graft dimensions. The neoseptum is then placed on top of the premaxillary DC-F graft and sutured to the ANS in the usual fashion.

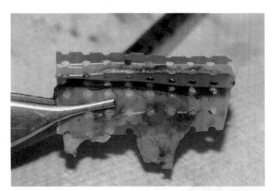

Fig. 12. Reconstruction of internal valve with folded PDS foil.

Reconstruction of the Internal Nasal Valves Using Polydioxanone Foil

Spreader grafts are usually preferred for widening of the internal nasal valves during extracorporeal septal reconstruction. Spreader flaps may also be used for reconstruction of the internal nasal valves, but spreader grafts are more effective at preventing skeletal destabilization after osteotomies. However, previous surgery or nasal trauma may have destroyed the surplus septal graft tissue necessitating spreader graft harvest from the concha or rib cage. In addition, because ear cartilage has suboptimal shape and because patients sometimes refuse rib graft harvest, we occasionally must use perforated 0.2 mm–thick PDS foil for internal valve reconstruction. Long narrow strips are first cut and sutured to the dorsal septum with the outer edge protruding slightly above the existing profile line. Next, the foil is folded outward (flush with the septal profile line) until a narrow shelf is created for suture reattachment of the ULCs. Owing to the springlike rigidity of the folded PDS foil, the junction of the ULC and dorsal septum is better supported for greater internal valve patency (**Fig. 12**).

RESULTS

Favorable long-term results are needed to validate the efficacy of any surgical technique. Although our initial experience with extracorporeal septoplasty revealed a high proportion of minor complications, clinical experience with more than 3000 extracorporeal septal reconstructions over a span of 3 decades has led to an evolution of our technique that has greatly reduced our initial complication rate. Even in the first 404 cases, in which close follow-up revealed frequent minor complications (**Table 1**), 96% of the patients having extracorporeal septoplasty still experienced good to excellent postoperative nasal airway

function.[11] Moreover, the most common complication observed in this series was irregularity of the dorsal contour (8.6%), but all of these patients were treated using the endonasal (closed) rhinoplasty approach in which secure suture fixation of the neoseptum is hindered by limited surgical exposure, which is in contrast with our current technique in which wide-field surgical exposure and transosseous suture fixation made possible by the external rhinoplasty approach have greatly reduced dorsal contour irregularities.[12] In addition, only one-third of the patients who developed a

Table 1 Complications of extracorporeal septal reconstruction	
Early	**N = 404**
Abscess of the dorsum	1
Septal perforation	1
Stitch visible through the skin	1
Immediate postoperative saddle nose	1
Epistaxis	2
Total	6 (1.5%)
Late	**N = 404**
Irregularities of the dorsum	35
Synechia	3
Dislocation of the septum	2
Total	40 (10%)
Other deformities independent from the septal reconstruction: deviation of the nasal pyramid	20 (5%)
Patients who thought revision surgery was worthwhile	16 (3%)
Revision surgery because of deviated nasal pyramid	3

postoperative dorsal irregularity (3.6% of the total) thought that the problem warranted revision surgery. This finding compares favorably to the medical literature, in which slightly more than 30% of patients required surgical revision after treatment with traditional septoplasty techniques.[13] It is worth noting that our initial septal slippage rate of 6.4% has also been decreased by half with the advent of transosseous suture fixation techniques.[14]

A variety of other minor complications were also observed in this early patient series.[11] One patient developed a postoperative dorsal abscess, which was drained and healed without further problems. A septal perforation was observed in 1 case, and a saddle-nose deformity developed in another. Two patients developed postoperative epistaxis, 1 with primary hypertension and the other with a hereditary coagulopathy. Several patients initially complained of stiffness in the upper lip, but this problem resolved spontaneously after 6 months in all cases. In addition, 1 patient treated with augmentation of the nasal spine required revision surgery for partial excision of the augmentation graft, and 3 patients developed postoperative synechiae.

Since our initial patient series, various modifications have been added to our technique in order to enhance both the safety and efficacy of extracorporeal septal reconstruction. The most important modification of our technique is the use of the open (external) rhinoplasty approach. By using the wide-field surgical exposure afforded by the open rhinoplasty approach to better access the nasal framework, suture fixation of the neoseptum to the ULC is more thorough and precise. The wide-field exposure also frequently permits drill hole placement within the nasal bones to permit transosseous suture fixation of the septal keystone area; a critical step in reestablishing stability of the dorsal L strut. The open rhinoplasty approach also permits transosseous suture fixation of the caudal septum to the ANS, which is performed in virtually every case to further enhance stability of the neoseptum. Wide-field exposure of the nasal dorsum also facilitates use of the electric drill. By using the Lindeman bur to create parallel medial osteotomies that are centered in the midline around the central ethmoid complex, contouring of the misshapen bony vault is better controlled and more effective. When desired, the Lindeman bur can also be used to widen the open roof for more aggressive narrowing of the ultrawide bony pyramid. Moreover, when combined with both transverse and lateral osteotomies using the percutaneous technique, the wide and/or deviated bony vault can be completely, but gently,

mobilized for more effective realignment of the deviated nasal axis. The use of percutaneous osteotomies has substantially reduced the incidence of bony comminution, which was previously seen in 5% of extracorporeal septorhinoplasty cases.[14] In addition, the electric drill can be used with the cylindrical bit to smooth minor skeletal contour irregularities for improved cosmetic outcomes. When skeletal imperfections cannot be completely eliminated, the use of camouflage techniques can also be used to further improve the surface contour, especially in patients with thin nasal skin. Our initial preference for dorsal camouflage was an onlay graft consisting of allogenic fascia lata, but we currently use FDC paste (when available) throughout the nasal framework for concealing minor contour irregularities. FDC paste is preferred rather than allogenic fascia lata for its reliability and superior affordability.

In 2011 we published a retrospective review of the 60 patients who underwent extracorporeal septal reconstruction under our care from 1980 to 1981.[15] An attempt to contact these patients was only partially successful. Thirty-four patients could not be located because of obsolete contact information, and 2 patients were deceased, but 24 patients were successfully located. Of these, 3 agreed to return for photodocumentation (**Figs. 13–15**) and the remaining 21 patients were interviewed by phone. All of the patients evaluated by phone interview were pleased with their current functional and cosmetic outcome. Of the 3 patients who returned for follow-up, 1 presented with a residual dorsal hump. Although the patient was not bothered by the cosmetic imperfection, the patient indicated that the hump developed within the first year postoperatively, suggesting that nasal dorsum may stabilize within 12 months of surgery, in contrast with tip surgery, in which many years may elapse before the final outcome is evident.

In our most recent study, we attempted to contact 235 patients, including 39 patients with cleft lip and palate, who underwent extracorporeal septal reconstruction under our care from 2005 to 2006.[12] Follow-up of 6 years was available for 196 patients. Fifteen patients (7.5%) required revision surgery during the 6-year follow-up period: 12 for correction of dorsal irregularities, including 8 patients who required partial removal of allogenic fascia lata secondary to overcorrection, and 3 patients who required revision osteotomies. In 8 patients, the septum was also revised. Dorsal overcorrection following the use of allogenic fascia lata for dorsal augmentation has also been observed in other patients, and we hypothesize that this may be related to excessive fluid retention

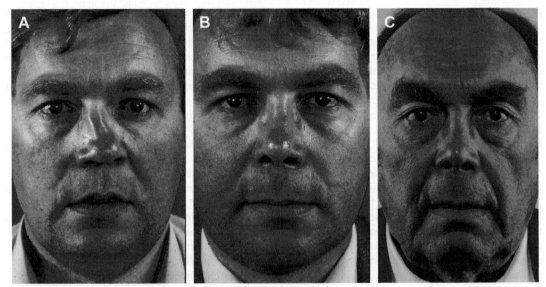

Fig. 13. Thirty-year follow-up of a patient undergoing extracorporeal septal reconstruction at the age of 36 years. (*A*) Before surgery, (*B*) 1 year after surgery, and (*C*) 30 years after surgery.

within the fascia, perhaps secondary to immersion of the fascia lata in antibiotic solution before implantation. Studies to elucidate the cause of this phenomenon are ongoing.

DISCUSSION

For more than 33 years we have been using extracorporeal septal reconstruction for the treatment of severe septal deformities. The concept of removing the septal partition for surgical correction outside of the nose was first published by King and

Ashley[1] in 1951, and later by Vilar-Sanch[16] (1984), Rees[6] (1986), and Jugo[5] (1987). We performed our first extracorporeal septal reconstruction in 1980 and have substantially modified our technique over the last 3 decades. The transition from the closed rhinoplasty approach to the open approach was a milestone in the evolution of our technique owing to a greater ease of dissection of the severely deformed septum, and to vastly improved stabilization of the reimplanted neoseptum; both direct consequences of wide-field surgical exposure. The advent of the external

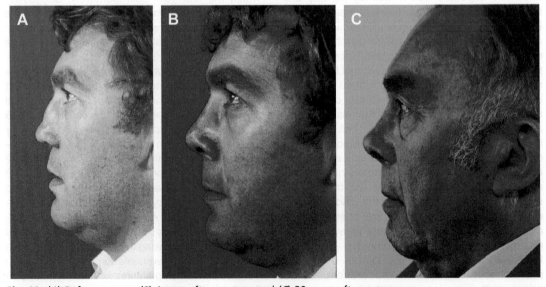

Fig. 14. (*A*) Before surgery, (*B*) 1 year after surgery, and (*C*) 30 years after surgery.

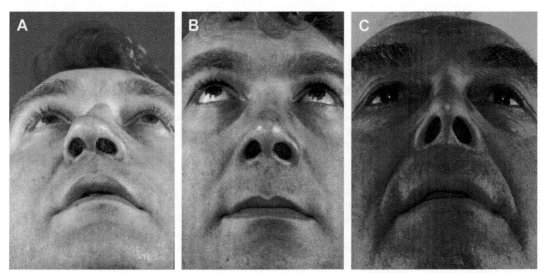

Fig. 15. (*A*) Before surgery, (*B*) 1 year after surgery, and (*C*) 30 years after surgery.

rhinoplasty approach allows even the novice surgeon to successfully treat severe septal deformities with favorable long-term results.

More recently, many other investigators have advocated using extracorporeal septoplasty, including D'Andrea and colleagues[17] (2011), Senyuva and colleagues[18] (1997), and Wilson and Mobley[19] (2011). However, others have advocated pseudoextracorporeal techniques in which the reconstruction is still performed in situ. Most[20] (2006) calls his anterior septal reconstruction a modified extracorporeal septoplasty, but this is just an exchange technique that is only possible if the dorsal strut is already straight. We still think that when a severe septal deformity involves the dorsal strut and/or the caudal septum it is better to remove the entire septal partition, preferably as a single piece, in order to reconstruct the L strut outside of the nose. In this manner, all of the tensions of the deformed septum can be isolated and eliminated individually to create a straight and stable skeletal framework. Unless all of the deformed portions of the septum are treated individually, the probability of treatment failure is unacceptably high, and most in situ techniques designed to straighten the caudal septum succeed only if the dorsal septum is already straight. In contrast, when both the dorsal and caudal segments of the L strut are severely deformed, in situ techniques are seldom effective and only extracorporeal techniques are likely to succeed. Concerns about permanently weakening the keystone area are unfounded because we routinely remove the keystone area as part of the initial septal resection, and secure long-term

anatomic reintegration of the neoseptum has been successful in most of our cases. Other clinicians have proposed modifications in which transosseous fixation of the caudal septum is omitted,[19] but we think that this comparatively simple and effective maneuver is an essential aspect of the treatment regimen. We therefore see no compelling reason to omit this step in fixation of the septal construct.

SUMMARY

Our clinical experience in more than 3000 patients treated since 1980 confirms the safety, efficacy, and reliability of extracorporeal septal reconstruction for the treatment of the severely twisted or deviated nose. Moreover, cosmetic and functional success rates exceeding 90% compare favorably with traditional septoplasty techniques, in which treatment failures are considerably higher.

ACKNOWLEDGMENT

I am very grateful to Rick Davis for helping me in translation and fruitfully discussing the issue.

REFERENCES

1. King ED, Ashley FL. The correction of internally and externally deviated nose. Plast Reconstr Surg 1952; 10:116–20.
2. Gubisch W. Aesthetic and functional reconstruction after nose trauma by septum replantation. Indian J Otolaryngol 1984;36:1–5.
3. Gubisch W. Zum problem der schiefnase. HNO NA 1988;2009–11.

4. Gubisch W. Das schwierige septum. HNO 1988;36: 286–9.
5. Jugo S. Total septal reconstruction through decortication (external) approach in children. Arch Otolaryngol Head Neck Surg 1987;13:173–86.
6. Rees TD. Surgical correction of the severely deviation nose by extramucosal excision of the osseocartilaginous septum and replacement as a free graft. Plast Reconstr Surg 1986;78(3):320–30.
7. Guyuron B. Rhinoplasty. New York: Elsvier; 2012. p. 307–9.
8. Gruber RP, Nahai F, Bogdan MA, et al. Changing the convexity and concavity of nasal cartilages and cartilage grafts with horizontal mattress sutures. Part II: clinical results. Plast Reconstr Surg 2005; 115:595.
9. Boenisch M, Nolst Trenite GJ. Reconstructive septal surgery. Facial Plast Surg 2006;22:249–54.
10. Daniel RK, Calvert JW. Diced cartilage grafts in rhinoplasty surgery. Plast Reconstr Surg 2003;113:2156.
11. Gubisch W. The extracorporeal septum plasty: a technique to correct difficult nasal deformities. Plast Reconstr Surg 1995;95:672–82.
12. Sommer C. Die extracorporale Septumrekonstruktion im Wandel. Wertigkeit und Risiko der extrakorporalen Septumrekonstruktion: Eine Studie an 264 Fällen. Inauguraldissertation de Medizinischen Fakultät Mannheim der Ruprecht-Karl-Universität Heidelberg. 2012.
13. Stal S. Septal deviation and correction of the crooked nose. In: Daniel RK, editor. Rhinoplasty. Boston: Little Brown; 1993.
14. Gubisch W. Septumplastik durch extrakorporale Korrektur. New York: Thieme Stuttgart; 1995.
15. Gubisch W. 30 years experience in extracorporeal septal reconstruction. Presented at 46th Annual Fall Meeting, AAFPS. San Francisco, September 8-11, 2011.
16. Vilar-Sancho B. Rhinoseptoplasty. Aesthetic Plast Surg 1984;8:61.
17. D'Andrea F, Grongo S, Rubino C. Extracorporeal septoplasty with paramarginal incision. Scand J Plast Reconstr Surg Hand Surg 2001;35(3):293–6.
18. Senyuva C, Yücel A, Aydin Y, et al. Extracorporeal septoplasty combined with open rhinoplasty. Aesthetic Plast Surg 1997;21(4):233–9.
19. Wilson MA, Mobley SR. Extracorporeal septoplasty: complications and new techniques. Arch Facial Plast Surg 2011;13(2):85–90.
20. Most SP. Anterior septal reconstruction. Arch Facial Plast Surg 2006;8:202.

Lateral Crural Tensioning for Refinement of the Wide and Underprojected Nasal Tip: Rethinking the Lateral Crural Steal

CrossMark

Richard E. Davis, MD[a,b],*

KEYWORDS

- Wide nasal tip • Lateral crural steal • Caudal septal extension graft • Tongue-in-groove setback
- Alar rim graft

KEY POINTS

- Excisional rhinoplasty techniques, such as the cephalic trim maneuver, often alter nasal tip size at the expense of structural stability.
- Effective refinement of the wide nasal tip does not mandate aggressive excision of the cephalic margin.
- The septal extension graft (SEG) creates a sturdy and stationary platform to allow precise positioning and suspension of the tip cartilage complex.
- The lateral crural steal (LCS) borrows from the overly long lateral crura to elongate the foreshortened medial crura to correct the alar cartilage length imbalance typical of the wide and underprojected nasal tip.
- In addition to cosmetic benefits of the traditional LCS, lateral crural tensioning (LCT) improves lower nasal sidewall tone and increases the threshold for dynamic nasal valve collapse by preserving the lateral crus and the nasal scroll and by stretching and tensioning the lateral crus.

BACKGROUND

Refining the overly wide nasal tip is among the most common, yet also among the most difficult, challenges in cosmetic rhinoplasty. Until recently, surgical strategies to reduce tip width have been largely dependent on cartilage excision for alterations in lobular size and shape. Despite the immediate and discernable reduction in nasal tip size, aggressive cartilage excision often fails to enhance tip contour in a controlled and predictable manner. As a consequence, aggressive excision-based techniques are increasingly recognized as haphazard, unpredictable, and disproportionately prone to undesirable postoperative contour deformities.[1–11] The outcome is frequently a nasal tip that is both unattractive and dysfunctional and one that usually deteriorates significantly over time (**Fig. 1**).

In response to the unacceptably high morbidity of aggressive excisional rhinoplasty techniques, most accomplished rhinoplasty surgeons have adopted strategies that preserve tip cartilage and/or augment skeletal tip support, thereby improving

No financial support or disclosures.
Conflicts of Interest: None.
a The Center for Facial Restoration, 1951 Southwest 172nd Avenue, Miramar, FL 33029, USA; b Division of Facial Plastic Surgery, Department of Otolaryngology - Head & Neck Surgery, University of Miami Miller School of Medicine, 1120 Northwest 14th Street, 5th Floor, Miami, FL 33136, USA
* The Center for Facial Restoration, 1951 Southwest 172nd Avenue, Miramar, FL 33029.
E-mail address: drd@davisrhinoplasty.com

Facial Plast Surg Clin N Am 23 (2015) 23–53
http://dx.doi.org/10.1016/j.fsc.2014.09.003
1064-7406/15/$ – see front matter © 2015 Elsevier Inc. All rights reserved.

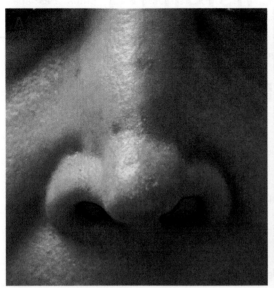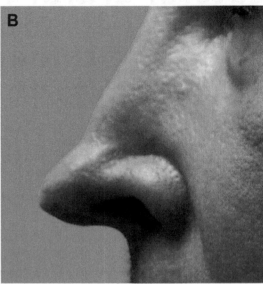

Fig. 1. Nasal tip deformity from lateral crural over-resection. Frontal (*A*) and left profile (*B*) views of a severely over-resected nasal tip with compromised skeletal support. Note lobular pinching, tip bossae, supra-alar pinching, alar retraction, and tip asymmetry.

long-term contour stability and airway patency.[1–15] Although this trend is rapidly spreading among rhinoplasty enthusiasts, the number of failed rhinoplasty outcomes stemming from cartilage over-resection seems to be growing rapidly, suggesting that aggressive excisional techniques are still practiced widely even today.[1] Nonetheless, there are now safe and effective alternatives to excisional rhinoplasty in which little if any tip cartilage excision is required. These techniques seek to preserve the existing tip cartilage and to alter tip contour via suture techniques, cartilage repositioning, and/or augmentation grafting to achieve an elegant and stable tip contour. And because the overly wide nasal tip is perhaps the most common morphology prompting cosmetic tip surgery, mastery of nonexcisional/structurally based rhinoplasty techniques is essential for the contemporary rhinoplasty surgeon.

The lateral crural steal (LSC) is the pejorative name given to an effective and tissue-conservative technique of nasal tip refinement. Resurrected in the contemporary rhinoplasty literature by Kridel and colleagues in 1989,[16] the traditional LCS achieves several cosmetic improvements with one comparatively simple surgical maneuver: relocation of the domal apices. Moreover, unlike excisional rhinoplasty techniques, the traditional LCS is not contingent on aggressive cartilage excision to achieve tip refinement. Instead, the LCS uses redistribution and/or repositioning of the existing skeletal elements to derive a more attractive,

stable, and functional tip configuration. Although a modest amount of cartilage must be excised from the nasal dome when performing an aggressive LCS, cartilage removal is confined to the medial-most aspect of the lateral crus in an area of comparatively minimal structural consequence,[11] thereby preserving virtually all of the naturally derived skeletal support. And, when the traditional LCS is used in combination with a SEG, the LCS/SEG combination—herein referred to as LCT—becomes a far more potent and versatile surgical workhorse for tip refinement.[1–3] With skillful execution, LCT not only achieves contour elegance with reliable long-term contour stability but also serves to protect or improve nasal valve patency.

The overly wide nasal tip is perhaps the most common tip malformation encountered in cosmetic nasal surgery. Although excess tip width may occur in isolation, it more commonly occurs in combination with inadequate tip projection and/or tip ptosis (ie, inadequate tip rotation). Historically, treatment of the wide, underprojected, and ptotic nasal tip—herein referred to as the compound tip deformity (CTD)—has been directed at volume reduction of the nasal tip cartilages. However, the CTD stems from more than just oversized tip cartilages, and volumetric reduction alone seldom achieves a satisfactory tip contour. Optimal refinement of the CTD necessitates correction of each anatomic malformation contributing to the unsightly tip morphology, not just volume reduction. For the CTD, excessive rounding of the nasal domes, excessive divergence of the nasal domes, and a length imbalance between the medial and lateral crura must all be corrected to achieve an elegant and natural-appearing tip contour. Rounding of the domal arches and excessive separation of the domal apices have both long been recognized as a major source of excessive lobular width,[17] even when alar cartilage length is normal. And when the transverse (vertical) height of the lateral crura is also excessive, additional lateral crural deformity, characterized by increased convexity of the entire crural span, exacerbates the

CTD by creating a wide supratip and/or an unsightly polly beak fullness of the supratip (**Fig. 2**). A less commonly recognized abnormality of the CTD, however, is the length imbalance between the medial and lateral crura created by medial displacement of the domal apices (ie, the tip defining points [TDPs]). Length discrepancies between the medial and lateral crura and their effects on positioning of the TDPs have been previously described by Adamson and colleagues[7] in their delineation of the M-Arch model of tip dynamics. In the healthy and attractive nasal tip, longitudinal

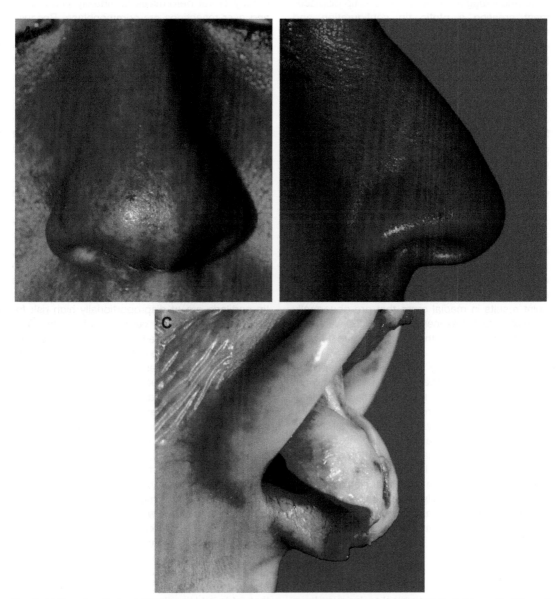

Fig. 2. CTD and polly beak fullness from convex cupping of wide lateral crura. Frontal (*A*), right profile (*B*), and intraoperative right profile (*C*) views. Note the cupped and overly wide lateral crura (*C*) contributing to excessive supratip width (*A*) and polly beak supratip fullness (*B*).

stiffness of the lateral crura thrusts the tip anteriorly and inferiorly. This is counterbalanced by the opposing anterior and superior thrust of the medial crura to create both equilibrium and stability within the lower lateral cartilage (LLC) arch. The equilibrium is further stabilized by the surrounding soft tissues. In the CTD, however, these relationships are anomalous. Although the *overall* length of the widened LLC arch is often normal or near normal, in the CTD, the nasal domes (and thus the TDPs) are skewed medially, resulting in abnormally long lateral crura and disproportionately short medial crura (**Fig. 3**). Overly long lateral crura bow outward and exaggerate the downward tip displacement creating a ptotic tip configuration and excessive width in the tip and supratip. In a review of 500 consecutive cases of nasal tip ptosis, Foda[18] found inferiorly oriented alar cartilages were the main cause of tip ptosis in 85% of patients presenting with a drooping tip. The CTD is also frequently exacerbated by pronounced convex cupping (ie, bulbosity) of the lateral crura, both longitudinally and transversely, which not only adds to lobular width but also dramatically increases supratip fullness (**Fig. 4**). Ironically, although bulbous cupping of the lateral crura increases crural stiffness, and therefore enhances lower nasal sidewall support, bulbosity also creates a highly objectionable cosmetic deformity that frequently prompts over-resection of the lateral crura and subsequent destabilization of the tip architecture. The anatomic counterpart to overly long lateral crura is overly short medial crura. Medial displacement of the domal breakpoint results in medial crura that are abnormally short and stubby, exacerbating the CTD with inadequate projection of the nasal tip (see **Fig. 3**). Moreover, inadequate tip projection is compounded by secondary splaying of the alar base, which further exacerbates the unsightly width deformity. Perhaps the most extreme example of alar cartilage maldistribution is the unilateral cleft-lip nasal deformity. In the unilateral cleft-lip nose, a severe ipsilateral length disparity between the foreshortened medial crus and the elongated lateral crus results from lateral, inferior, and posterior displacement of the ipsilateral alar base. This developmental deformity is best corrected by repositioning the ectopic alar base and redistributing the malformed LLC with a unilateral LCS-type domal repositioning.[19]

THE CEPHALIC TRIM

Historically, a variety of surgical techniques have been advocated for refinement of the overly wide nasal tip. Perhaps the least effective technique for tip refinement is the cephalic trim maneuver. The cephalic trim maneuver seeks to simultaneously narrow, refine, and rotate the ptotic and overly wide nasal tip simply by resecting the cephalic margin of both lateral crural cartilages. In theory, precise and judicious trimming of the cephalic margin strategically weakens the lateral crura leading to a refined and slightly rotated nasal tip,[20] but only if the volume and location of the excised crural cartilage correspond perfectly to the required distribution and degree of structural weakening. In reality, determining how much cartilage can be safely excised without triggering secondary crural deformities is virtually impossible, and over-resections are commonplace. Because the average lateral crus measures only approximately 12 mm in (vertical) width,[21,22] even the generally accepted residual crural width of 6.0 mm preserves only approximately half of the original crural height. Furthermore, because lateral crural thickness averages only 0.7 mm,[22] resecting half of the crural height often results in a narrow and flimsy crural remnant that is incapable of supporting either the nasal tip or the lower nasal sidewall. Because LLC stiffness is a primary component of tip contour and support,[23] an over-aggressive cephalic resection can destabilize the tip architecture with disastrous consequences. The eventual result is often severe distortion of the nasal tip leading to lobular pinching, alar retraction, bossae formation, asymmetry, excessive tip rotation, unwanted loss of tip projection, and/or symptomatic nasal valve collapse.[1–12,20,24,25] Patients with naturally weak tip cartilage are at disproportionally high risk for morbidity after the cephalic trim maneuver because the tip is already at or near the threshold for collapse, and these patients often develop unsightly tip deformities despite comparatively modest cephalic resections.[1–3,24] Moreover, tip width does not correlate with cartilage stiffness, and overly pliable, weak tip cartilages are often encountered in ultrawide bulbous noses.[1–3] Ironically, the combination of weak tip cartilage and a comparatively severe cosmetic deformity often prompts overzealous treatment and subsequent tip deformity. Similarly, over-resection of the cephalic margin is also more likely to distort the tip architecture in noses with extremes of skin thickness. In the thin-skinned nose, shrink-wrap contracture is often forceful and sustained, leading to a higher incidence of bossae, buckling, and alar retraction. However, the morbidity of over-resection is also exacerbated by ultrathick skin that adds additional weight to the frail and surgically dilapidated tip framework (**Fig. 5**).[4,7,11,26] Ironically, severe crural over-resection may not

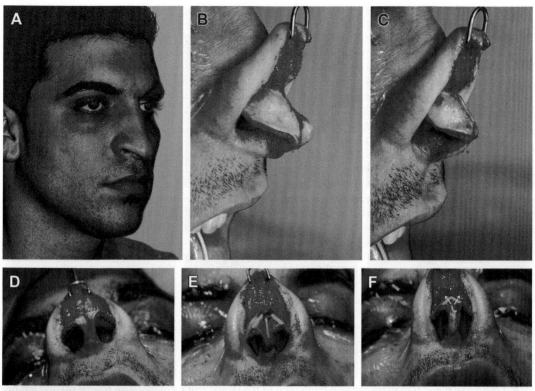

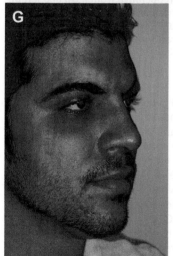

Fig. 3. Medial and lateral crural length discrepancy from malposition of the domal apex. Preoperative right oblique view (*A*) demonstrating overly long lateral crura with severe tip ptosis, and overly short medial crura with inadequate tip projection. Intraoperative right oblique view (*B*) demonstrating the crural length discrepancy. Intraoperative right oblique view (*C*) after LCS to correct crural length imbalance. Note alteration in length of the lateral and medial crura. Intraoperative base views demonstrating underprojected alar cartilages before treatment (*D*), formation of the neodomes with domal folds (*blue lines*) oriented perpendicular to the long axis of the lateral crus to preserve infratip divergence (*E*), and completed LCS after suture approximation of the neodomes to conceal the SEG (*F*). Note persistent divergence of the domal folds (*blue lines*) at completion of the LCS, and the oblique direction of suture passage (*yellow arrows*). Postoperative right oblique view (*G*) demonstrating a natural and attractive tip contour using the LCS technique.

become immediately evident in the thick-skinned nose because postoperative swelling—which is typically more severe and longer lasting in thick nasal skin—may conceal the initial tip deformity for many months. However, as the swelling subsides and the surgically weakened tip framework is subjected to the sustained and potent forces of fibrosis combined with the repetitive inward sidewall flexion generated during nasal inspiration, stigmatic tip deformities and/or functional impairment eventually become evident. Finally, even when the cephalic trim fails to initially exceed the threshold for skeletal collapse, age or disease-related deterioration in crural stiffness may also lead to eventual tip deformities, particularly because many surgeons fail to account for future losses in cartilage strength when planning crural resections. Although tip suturing techniques are now commonly used in combination with the cephalic trim for tip refinement, the inappropriate or overzealous use of tip sutures can themselves cause postsurgical tip deformities, and aggressive

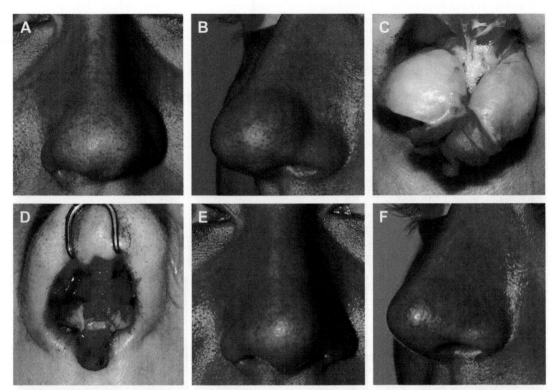

Fig. 4. Longitudinal and transverse cupping (bulbosity) of the lateral crura. Preoperative frontal (*A*) and left oblique views (*B*) demonstrating pronounced bulbosity of the alar cartilages, intraoperative frontal views revealing bulbous and asymmetric tip cartilages (*C*) reconfigured tip cartilages after LCT, cephalic turn-in flaps, bilateral AARGs (double on right side), and shield graft placement (*D*), and postoperative frontal (*E*) left oblique views (*F*) demonstrating elimination of tip bulbosity.

resections of the cephalic margin usually serve to increase the likelihood of such problems.[1-3,6-8] Owing to the synergistic and destabilizing triad of (1) surgically compromised structural support, (2) chronic deformational forces of wound healing, and (3) age-related losses in cartilage strength, the adverse effects of crural over-resection frequently worsen for decades, making the cephalic trim a risky undertaking associated with considerable long-term morbidity in susceptible patients. And when crural over-resection is combined with over-resection of the anterior nasal septum, which undergirds and supports the tip complex, virtually all of the adverse consequences of the cephalic trim are intensified.[1-4,27]

OVERLY LONG LATERAL CRURA—A FREQUENTLY NEGLECTED DEFORMITY

Treating the constellation of LLC deformities that characterizes the CTD—in particular, the overly wide tip cartilages and the abnormalities of domal shape and spacing—has improved greatly in the past 3 decades. Structural techniques that enhance skeletal support for improved contour stability and nondestructive suture-based techniques that reshape and reposition malformed or malpositioned tip cartilages have transformed the quality and long-term predictability of tip rhinoplasty.[1-10,12-18] Over this same time period, however, comparatively little attention has been directed at another important anatomic deformity common to the CTD: the crural length disparity that results from malposition of the nasal domes. Despite the adverse impact on tip aesthetics, maldistribution of tip cartilage is a critical aberration of tip architecture that can dramatically affect lobular contour, supratip contour, tip support, sidewall aesthetics, and nasal valve function, yet one that is often overlooked, undertreated, and/or mismanaged. And although placement of a columellar strut graft or an SEG enhances central tip support by augmenting medial crural length, such techniques alone fail to treat the corresponding excess in lateral crural length that results from malposition of the apical fold. The persistent excess length of the lateral crura coupled with their caudally directed forces of tip displacement may explain

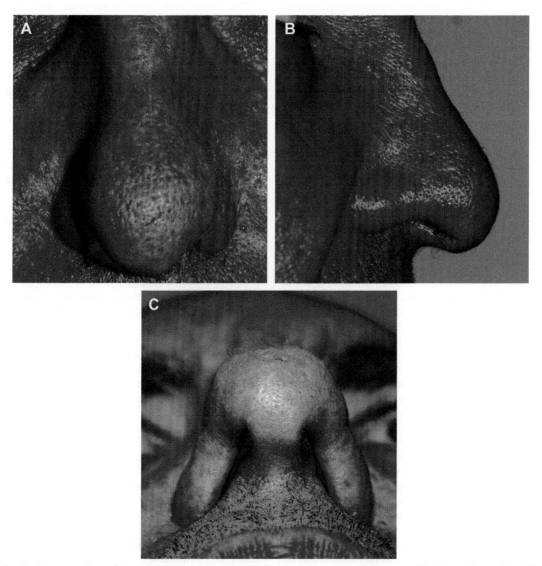

Fig. 5. Over-resection of the lateral crura in an ultrathick skinned nose. Frontal (*A*), profile (*B*), and base views (*C*) after subtotal resection of the lateral crura (performed elsewhere) in a middle-aged man with ultrathick nasal skin. Note severe external valve collapse and tip ptosis from compromised skeletal support. According to the patient, the collapse developed gradually several months after surgery.

the failure of columellar strut grafts to consistently maintain tip projection.[28] Similarly, the unrecognized crural length surplus may also explain the continued use of overaggressive cephalic resections in a misguided and ill-fated attempt to eliminate unwanted supratip fullness. And when over-resection of the oversized lateral crus does occur, a flail segment usually ensues because the excess crural length remains unreconciled. Although some surgeons have advocated lateral crural overlap (LCO) techniques, in which the lateral crura are divided vertically, overlapped by several millimeters to reduce crural length, and then reattached with mattress sutures,[7,18,29,30]

vertical sectioning of the alar cartilage, although effective at truncating crural length, reduces tip projection and potentially destabilizes the lateral crural span – both consequences that can be avoided entirely with the use of the LCS. Moreover, in a 500-patient (consecutive) series comparing the standard LCS and the LCO technique for treatment of the ptotic and underprojected nasal tip, the LCS was deemed preferable because tip projection and rotation were both increased simultaneously.[18] This confirmed findings of previous work in which the LCS was preferred over the LCO for simultaneous increases in tip projection and tip rotation.[30] Regardless of the preferred treatment method, excessive lateral crural length is an often-ignored yet fundamental anomaly of the CTD that has a profound impact on form and function of the nasal base; and failure to shorten the overly long lateral crus while maintaining the structural integrity of the lateral crural span inevitably taints an otherwise satisfactory surgical outcome.

SIDEWALL TENSION—THE UNRECOGNIZED BENEFIT OF THE LATERAL CRURAL STEAL

Unlike the cephalic trim technique, which sacrifices natural skeletal support and ignores the crural length discrepancy, thereby converting a wide and overly prominent lateral crural span into a collapsed and flail segment vulnerable to distortion from scar contracture, the traditional LCS restores balanced and aesthetically pleasing crural proportions by lengthening the undersized medial crura at the expense of the overly long lateral crura (**Fig. 6**). The redistribution of tip cartilage is accomplished without excising large segments of the cephalic margin or vertically dividing the LLC but simply by relocating the natural domal fold (or apex) that establishes the breakpoint between the medial and lateral crus and which delineates the TDP. Relocating the domal fold and creating a neodome results in several simultaneous functional and cosmetic benefits.[1–3,16,18,30] First, as the relocated nasal domes are approximated in the midline, tip width is substantially reduced. Spacing of the neodomes and acuity of the domal angles can also be independently adjusted with tip sutures to fine-tune lobular width according to variations in skin thickness and cosmetic preferences. Second, neodomal approximation also simultaneously increases both tip rotation and tip projection as the length imbalance between the medial and lateral crura is eliminated. Thus, with a single nondestructive maneuver, the traditional LCS addresses all 3 major cosmetic abnormalities of the CTD—excessive lobular width, tip ptosis, and inadequate tip projection. And because each neodome is constructed independently, modest preexisting asymmetries in domal arch projection and/or tip rotation can be offset with differential dome positioning. Finally, when the LCS is used for aggressive increases in tip projection, a secondary reduction in nasal base width often occurs as an additional cosmetic benefit of alar cartilage redistribution.

One of the most important but unrecognized benefits of an aggressive LCS involves secondary improvements in nasal tip dynamics. As the neodomes are suture approximated in the midline, longitudinal tensioning forces are generated that stretch and tighten both lateral crura. Unlike many other contemporary tip refinement strategies that rely on bulky structural grafts, such as the lateral crural strut graft (LCSG)[31] or the crural batten graft,[32] to contour and support the lax lower nasal sidewall (with or without cephalic resection), the LCT approach to tip refinement exploits the tensioning forces generated from tip refinement to increase crural rigidity and subsequently to strengthen and contour the lower nasal sidewall.[1–3] And because lateral crural augmentation grafts are frequently obviated, limited graft materials are conserved, and the additional weight and mass effect of structural grafts can be avoided. Because LCT also shortens and tightens the lateral crura without the need for cephalic resection, the entire nasal scroll and its sizable contribution to sidewall support are also preserved. And because the nasal scroll lies at the epicenter of the internal nasal valve—a dynamic flow-regulating apparatus that is sensitive to even minor reductions in cross-sectional area resulting from bulky sidewall grafts or crural over-resection—the nondestructive LCT maneuver is far less likely to disrupt nasal airflow. Moreover, additional cosmetic enhancements are also derived from LCT. Because the lateral crura are tethered laterally at the piriform aperture, tensioning forces created by LCT also stretch and flatten the lateral crura with a noticeable reduction in crural convexity and bulbosity, particularly in patients with weak tip cartilage.[1–3] The result of this sidewall tensioning effect is a more slender and elegant supra-tip contour, accompanied by a concomitant increase in resting sidewall tone and a corresponding increase in the threshold for dynamic nasal valve collapse. Hence, unlike most other contemporary strategies for treating the CTD, the LCT approach also simultaneously enhances nasal valve physiology by (1) preserving virtually all of the existing natural skeletal support, (2) eliminating laxity derived from excess lateral crural length, and (3) increasing lower nasal sidewall tone with tensioning forces—all without the use of lateral crural augmentation grafts. In previously operated noses presenting with concave sagging of the lower nasal sidewall from lateral crural over-resection, the tensioning forces generated by LCT also serve to lift and tighten flail crural segments, thereby minimizing unsightly sidewall pinching while dramatically enlarging internal nasal valve dimensions.[1–3] Similarly, sidewall tensioning can also be used to prevent and/or minimize alar retraction. In primary rhinoplasty, stretching and tightening of the lateral crura with LCT not only flattens the crura but also

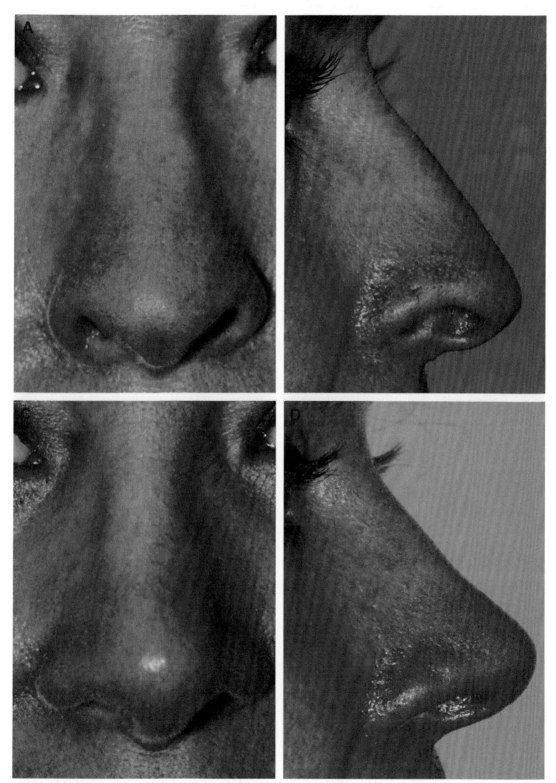

Fig. 6. Cosmetic benefits of the LCT technique. Preoperative frontal (*A*) and profile (*B*) views demonstrating a wide and underprojected tip with congenital alar retraction. Postoperative frontal (*C*) and profile (*D*) views demonstrating an improved columellar-alar relationship with simultaneous improvements in lobular width, tip projection, and tip rotation.

creates a guitar string effect that opposes upward displacement from scar contracture. And because sidewall tensioning generally obviates a traditional cephalic trim, preservation of the full vertical height of the lateral crus further buttresses the alar rim against vertical scar contracture. In the over-resected tip presenting with iatrogenic alar retraction, sidewall tensioning, combined with lysis of cephalic adhesions and unfurling of the contracted internal lining, can

stabilize the repositioned crural remnant against recurrent retraction (**Fig. 7**), particularly if the crural remnant is also further supported with modified alar rim grafts.[1–3] Although severe alar retraction may require more-aggressive techniques to stabilize the alar rim, such as the LCSG,[31] with or without lateral crural repositioning,[33] aggressive sidewall tensioning alone is sufficient in a large percentage of cases. However, the use of LCT does not preclude the combined

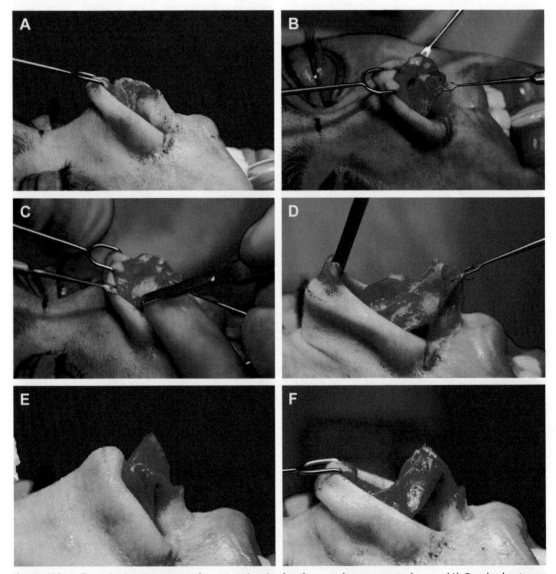

Fig. 7. Sidewall tensioning to correct alar retraction in the short and over-resected nose. (*A*) Overly short nose after overzealous excisional rhinoplasty. (*B*) Counterrotation of lateral crural (remnants) prevented by fibrous adhesion of the cephalic margin. (*C*) Sharp lysis of fibrous adhesions to unfurl contracted vestibular skin and release retracted lateral crura. (*D*) Improved tip cartilage mobility after lysis of fibrous adhesions. (*E*) Placement of SEG to reproject, counterrotate, and tension the lateral crural remnants. (*F*) Counterrotated and reprojected tip cartilage after fixation to SEG.

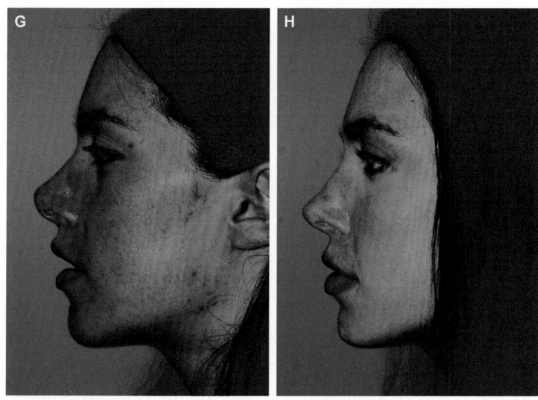

Fig. 7. (*continued*) Sidewall tensioning to correct alar retraction in the short and over-esected nose. (*G*) Pre-operative lateral view. (*H*) 1-year post-operative lateral view. (*From* Davis RE. Revision rhinoplasty. In: Johnson JT, Rosen CA, editors. Bailey's Head and Neck Surgery – Otolaryngology. 5th edition. Philadelphia, Baltimore (MD), New York: Wolters Kluwer/Lippincott; Williams, & Wilkins; 2014. p. 3017; with permission.)

use of the LCSG for the treatment of severe alar retraction, and because the mechanisms of alar rim stabilization are compatible with LCT, the combined use of LCT and LCSG is likely to be more effective, albeit with a greater risk of internal nasal valve impingement from LCSG bulk. In summary, LCT mimics the natural dynamics of an attractive and fully functional nasal sidewall by stiffening the existing crural cartilage and raising the threshold for dynamic internal valve collapse, all while maintaining a thin, lightweight, and flexible nasal sidewall—a particularly useful benefit when treating the long and ultraslender nose where LCSGs may compromise internal valve patency, efface the supra-alar crease, and/or partially restrict mimetic movement.[1–3,34] LCT also expands the already potent cosmetic benefits of the traditional LCS by flattening the entire lateral crus to eliminate unsightly fullness of the supratip. Hence, by reallocating and reshaping the LLC using almost entirely reversible suture techniques, LCT can custom-contour the CTD while enhancing or preserving airway function and reducing the dependence on large structural grafts.

INCREASING POTENCY OF THE LATERAL CRURAL STEAL WITH THE SEPTAL EXTENSION GRAFT

Although the classic LCS can simultaneously narrow, project, and rotate a wide, underprojected, and ptotic nasal tip, recruiting more than a few millimeters of the lateral crura usually results in over-rotation of the nasal tip and excessive nostril show. To prevent tip over-rotation and excessive nostril show, the newly configured tip complex must be firmly stabilized against unwanted cephalic and/or posterior displacement.[1–3] Although the conventional columellar strut graft is effective at stabilizing the tip against unwanted deprojection, it does little to prevent over-rotation after an aggressive LCS. Because recruiting large amounts of lateral crural cartilage inevitably leads to increasingly powerful forces of tip rotation,[35] these forces can easily displace an unsupported tip/columellar strut complex in an upward (cephalad) direction. Consequently, it is essential to combine an aggressive LCS with an SEG to prevent unwanted tip rotation and stabilize tip positioning. The SEG is a modified columellar strut graft that is sutured to the caudal septum to enhance stability of the tip complex and is especially useful after large increases in nasal length and/or tip projection.[28,36–40] By securing the SEG to the caudal L-strut, a stationary and invisible support column—buttressed indirectly from above by the bony facial skeleton—is created to suspend and immobilize the newly configured tip cartilages and to prevent excessive rotation triggered by aggressive lateral crural recruitment.[1–3] In essence, the SEG creates a tent pole effect that projects the skin envelope outward while opposing the upward pull generated by aggressive sidewall tensioning. Without the stationary fixation point generated by SEG placement, LCT is ill advised, and nearly all the cosmetic and functional benefits of nasal sidewall tensioning are rendered impossible. However, by fabricating an SEG of appropriate dimension and shape, precise 3-D positioning of the tip complex is limited only by availability of donor graft material and distensibility of the skin envelope. A properly crafted and sturdy SEG not only counters the forces of tip displacement generated by an aggressive LCT but also stretches a thick, fibrotic, and noncompliant skin envelope and resists distortion generated by excessive postoperative swelling. Although stabilization grafts, such as extended spreader grafts or splinting grafts, are occasionally necessary to prevent rudder-like deflection of the SEG and/or flexion of the dorsal L-strut in cases of high closing tension,[38–40] in noses with a readily distensible skin envelope, a properly secured SEG—further stabilized by suture fixation of the medial crura—facilitates significant increases in tip projection and/or nasal lengthening without the need for stabilization grafts (**Fig. 8**). In cases that do require stabilization grafts, encroachment of the internal nasal valve is more likely with bilateral extended spreader grafts—particularly in an ultraslender nose where even modest valve impingement can lead to symptomatic airway dysfunction—and stabilization is often best achieved using thin (unilateral) osseous splinting grafts fabricated from perforated segments of ethmoid or vomerine bone (**Fig. 9**). Extended spreader grafts, however, which are usually fashioned from rib cartilage, are well suited to the wide nose where nasal valve impingement is unlikely, and they are sometimes the only effective means for distending rigid and nondistensible nasal skin when re-expanding the severely over-resected nose. Although comparatively little donor cartilage is required to create an SEG, a stiff, flat, and slender graft is mandatory, and septal cartilage is preferred owing to its ideal shape and rigidity. However, when septal donor tissue is depleted or rendered unsuitable, a double-layered conchal cartilage graft or a rib cartilage graft can also be used effectively, albeit with additional graft thickness. Finally, in exchange for the unparalleled benefits of the SEG, a permanently stiff and rigid tip complex is inevitable. Although the fully healed tip still flexes easily from side to side, the ability to compress the tip complex is permanently lost. Although tip rigidity is sometimes cited as a contraindication to SEG use owing to patient nonacceptance, after nearly 2 decades of SEG use, the author has found nearly all patients readily accepting of this minor side effect of tip refinement.

PREOPERATIVE PREPARATIONS

All patients undergo a detailed preoperative medical screening history. Comorbidities, medications, or behaviors that may have an impact on safe and effective general anesthesia or that may impair wound healing are specifically sought. Details of any previous nasal surgery are also elicited. Physical examination is used to assess the nasal tissue characteristics, such as skin thickness and elasticity, cartilage stiffness, tip and sidewall support, septal alignment, previous septal cartilage excision, nasal valve patency and function, turbinate size, and the extent of previous surgical scarring. A careful elucidation of a patient's cosmetic objectives and standard preoperative photographs are also obtained. Computer imaging is also performed to determine optimal changes in tip projection, rotation, and width. Platelet inhibitors, such as aspirin-containing medications, nonsteroidal antiinflammatory drugs, herbal supplements, vitamin E, and omega fish oils, are discontinued at least 10 days prior to surgical treatment, and all smokers are advised to discontinue all forms of nicotine use at least 6 weeks prior to surgery. When appropriate, preoperative laboratory testing is also conducted based on previously established medical guidelines for preanesthesia testing.[41,42] In patients working as health care providers and in patients with a past history of methicillin-resistant *Staphylococcus aureus* infection, mupirocin ointment is applied to the vestibular skin twice daily for 5 days immediately prior to surgical treatment.

SURGICAL TECHNIQUE

Use of the LCT technique requires the open (external) rhinoplasty approach. Careful en bloc degloving of the skin/soft tissue envelope is performed in a subperichondrial/subperiosteal dissection plane to prevent unnecessary trauma

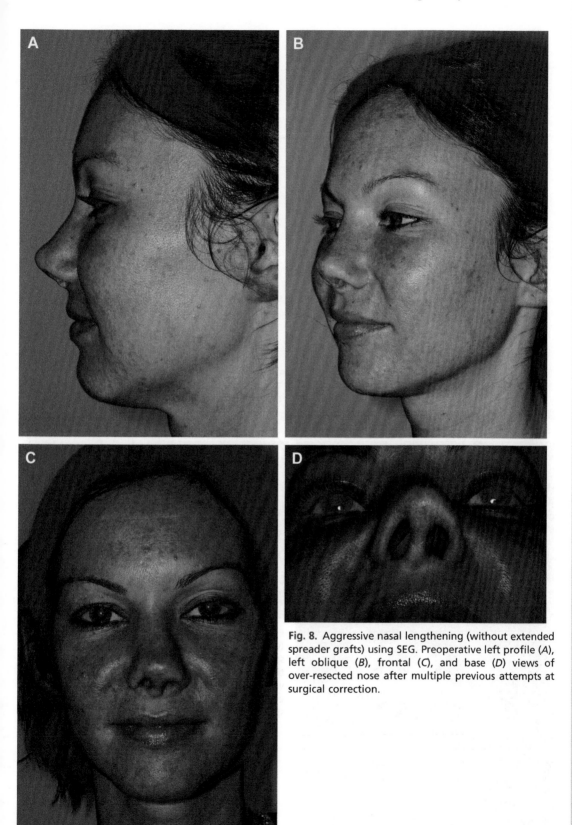

Fig. 8. Aggressive nasal lengthening (without extended spreader grafts) using SEG. Preoperative left profile (*A*), left oblique (*B*), frontal (*C*), and base (*D*) views of over-resected nose after multiple previous attempts at surgical correction.

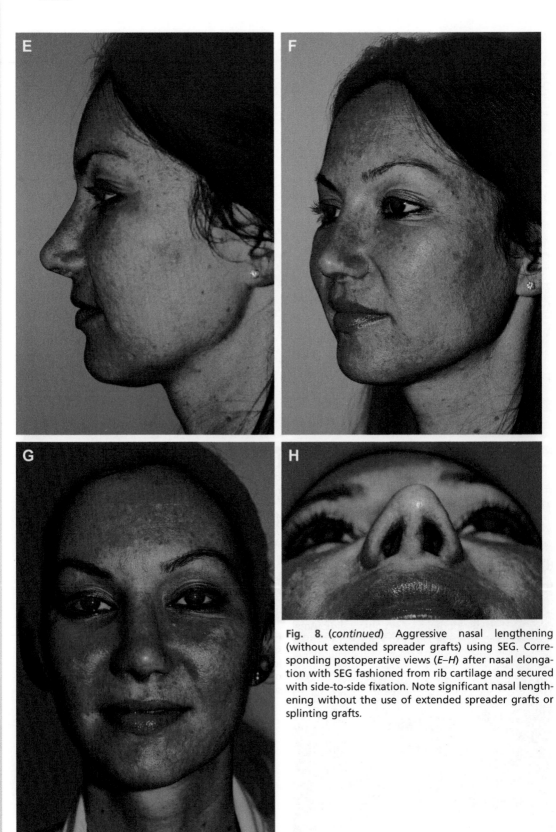

Fig. 8. (*continued*) Aggressive nasal lengthening (without extended spreader grafts) using SEG. Corresponding postoperative views (*E–H*) after nasal elongation with SEG fashioned from rib cartilage and secured with side-to-side fixation. Note significant nasal lengthening without the use of extended spreader grafts or splinting grafts.

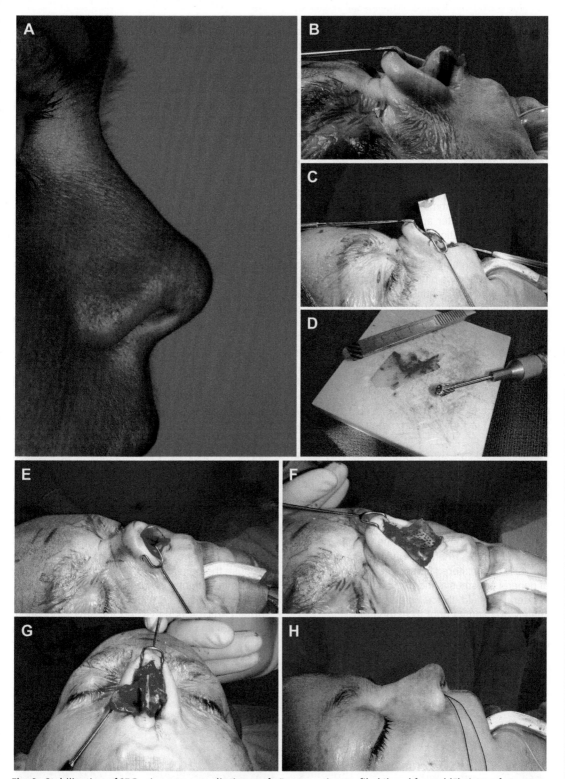

Fig. 9. Stabilization of SEG using osseous splinting graft. Preoperative profile (*A*) and frontal (*B*) views of a congenitally short nose with excessive nostril show. Intraoperative views of untreated cartilage (*C*), tracing of caudal septum for template creation (*D*), septal graft and cutting bur to thin septal bone during splinting graft fabrication (*E*), cartilaginous SEG secured in end-to-end alignment using figure-of-8 sutures (*F*), perforated vomerine splinting graft bridging the SEG and caudal septum from profile (*G*) and base (*H*) views (note thin graft profile on base view), and immediate postoperative views showing tip counter-rotation and decreased nostril show.

to the overlying subdermal vascular plexus. Controlled hypotension in young and healthy rhinoplasty patients (with a target mean arterial pressure of 60–65 mm Hg) is also used to minimize intraoperative bleeding, swelling, and ecchymosis and is most easily accomplished using general endotracheal anesthesia. Local anesthesia is initiated with topical anesthetization of the nasal mucosa using cotton pledgets saturated with 4% cocaine solution. Topical anesthetization of the nasal cavity improves visualization for local anesthetic infiltration and simultaneously eliminates most of the painful stimuli associated with subsequent injections. After approximately 10 minutes, topical anesthetization is followed by soft tissue infiltration of the outer nose and nasal airway using 1% lidocaine containing 1:100,000 epinephrine. In addition to muting painful stimuli, local anesthetic infiltration with epinephrine-containing solution is used to create a comparatively bloodless surgical field frequently obviating electrocautery. A total of approximately 3.0 mL of local anesthetic is first used to infiltrate the columella, tip, and the nasal sidewalls at the nasofacial groove. Direct infiltration of the dorsum is avoided to minimize contour distortion. Approximately, 4.0 to 9.0 mL of additional local anesthesia is then used to infiltrate the septum (and inferior turbinates when appropriate). Care is taken to administer local anesthesia gradually to prevent hemodynamic instability. Because local anesthesia eliminates nearly all intraoperative pain, narcotics are withheld throughout the entire procedure to reduce the risk of postoperative nausea and vomiting (PONV). To further reduce the risk of emesis, 4 mg of intravenous (IV) dexamethasone sodium phosphate (APP Pharmaceuticals, Schaumburg, Illinois) is administered immediately after induction of general anesthesia and 4 mg of IV ondansetron (Baxter, Deerfield, Illinois) is administered approximately 30 minutes prior to extubation.[43,44]

Prior to infiltration with local anesthesia, reference marks are made on the facial skin at the radix, at the TDPs (ie, the point of maximum tip projection), and at the columellar-labial junction. Preoperative baseline measurements of tip projection (at the TDP) (**Fig. 10**A) and nasal length (as determined by the distance between the radix and the TDP) (see **Fig. 10**B) are obtained prior to anesthetic infiltration and the values are recorded for later comparison. Tip projection is measured using a projectometer (Anthony Products, Indianapolis, Indiana) placed on the upper central incisor teeth and the forehead (see **Fig. 10**A). Positioning of the projectometer on the forehead skin is also marked for the consistency of subsequent measurements.

After complete degloving of the LLC (from the medial crural footpods to the sesamoid cartilages), the membranous septum is separated with sharp dissection to expose the caudal margin of the quadrangular cartilage. Complete (bilateral) exposure of the caudal septum and nasal spine (in the subperichondrial/subperiosteal plane) is performed to facilitate SEG placement, particularly if a tongue-in-groove (TIG) setback is also planned. The upper lateral cartilages (ULCs) are then degloved laterally to the piriform aperture for complete exposure of the cartilaginous nasal framework. Wide-field exposure is particularly important when performing LCT to optimize lateral crural mobilization and recruitment (**Fig. 11**). Although the extent of lateral crural recruitment varies from patient to patient, up to 7 to 8 mm of LCS can be achieved in some noses after the wide-field release of the skin/soft tissue envelope. Care is taken to elevate the outer soft tissue envelope in a symmetric fashion to minimize asymmetries derived from wound healing. In contrast to the outer skin envelope, however, the internal nasal lining is usually not dissected from the lateral crura because the benefits of LCT are derived in part by concomitant tightening of the vestibular lining.

After soft tissue degloving of the outer nose, septal cartilage is harvested for SEG fabrication. Care is taken to preserve a sturdy L-strut remnant because a rigid and flat L-strut is essential for

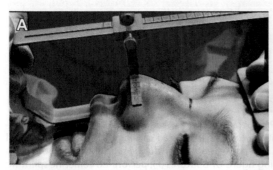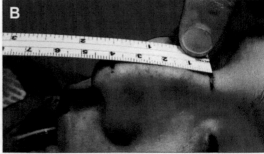

Fig. 10. Preoperative baseline tip measurements. (*A*) Measurement of preoperative tip projection using projectometer. (*B*) Measurement of preoperative TDP position relative to radix reference mark.

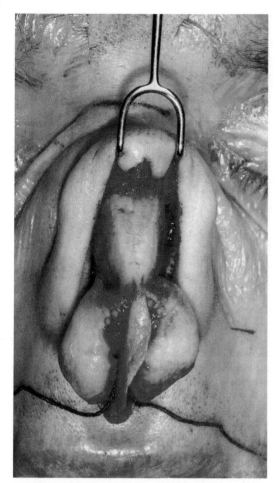

Fig. 11. Wide-field nasal dissection for complete release of the outer nasal soft tissue/skin envelope. Note full degloving of the cartilaginous framework just medial to the piriform aperture.

structural stability and effectiveness of the SEG bulwark. Hence, only cartilage essential to grafting objectives (or for treatment of nasal airway obstruction) is removed. Septal cartilage is reserved for the fabrication of the SEG and alar rim grafts, whereas alternative cartilage graft materials from the concha or rib cage are used for spreader grafting or for dorsal augmentation when sufficient amounts of septal cartilage are unavailable. In those patients needing large amounts of septal graft tissue, the natural stiffness of dorsal septum must be taken into consideration when determining residual L-strut size. A much wider L-strut should be retained in patients with weak septal cartilage unless compensatory techniques, such as spreader graft placement and/or osseous splinting of the dorsal L-strut, are also performed. In patients with unacceptably weak septal cartilage, it is often necessary to harvest secondary

sources of donor cartilage or autologous septal bone to augment L-strut rigidity and support. Perforated ethmoid or vomerine bone is an effective (autologous) alternative to septal cartilage for strengthening a weak or distorted L-strut when septal cartilage is unavailable. When using osseous splinting grafts, a pear-shaped cutting bur (Stryker, Kalamazoo, Michigan) is usually needed to create a thin and flat bony plate. The graft is then carefully perforated with numerous 1.0-mm drill holes to facilitate suture fixation and vascular in-growth (see **Fig. 9**). Regardless of the source of donor graft tissue, a straight and rigid dorsal septum is paramount.

In patients presenting with an ultrawide nasal tip and normal (or increased) tip projection, using the LCT approach to tip refinement inevitably results in lobular overprojection from aggressive lateral crural recruitment. Even traditional tip-narrowing sutures can alone produce modest degrees of overprojection in this circumstance.[1–3,6,7] Consequently, to prevent excess tip projection, LCT is preceded by a variation of the classic TIG setback, as previously described by Kridel and colleagues.[45] Unlike the classic technique in which the medial crura are moved in a mostly cephalad direction to shorten the nose, however, the modified TIG setback is used to initially underproject the tip/columellar complex by moving the medial crura inferiorly. The repositioned medial crura are then secured to the anterior nasal spine using percutaneous transfixion sutures of 4-0 poliglecaprone (Ethicon, Somerville, NJ, USA) passed through (transverse) osseous drill holes. In addition to immobilizing the medial crura, suture fixation permits narrowing of the columellar pedestal when desired. Initial underprojection of the ultrawide nasal tip complex is uniquely advantageous because it opens the door for a more aggressive LCT and thus better tip refinement, while simultaneously restoring tip projection to an acceptable level. And in overly long noses, or noses with an overly obtuse nasolabial angle or a hanging columella, the TIG setback can also be used to simultaneously shorten a long nose, deepen an obtuse nasolabial angle, and/or correct a hanging columella for further improvements in nasal base profile aesthetics (**Fig. 12**).[45,46] Because the combined TIG/LCS/SEG technique works to reposition and reconfigure the entire length of the LLC arch, tip refinement and nasal base profile aesthetics are both optimized, and unwanted increases in tip projection are avoided without negating the traditional benefits of LCS. Although the TIG setback is indispensable for reducing tip projection and/or enhancing nasal base profile aesthetics, it should be used judiciously when

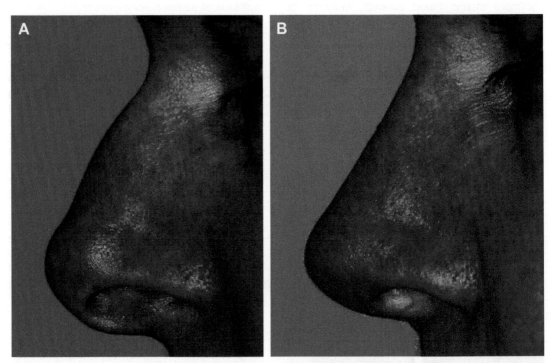

Fig. 12. Concomitant use of TIG setback to eliminate caudal excess and improve nasal base profile aesthetics. (*A*) Preoperative profile view demonstrating caudal excess nasal base deformity. (*B*) Postoperative profile view demonstrating improved nasal base contour after TIG setback combined with LCT technique.

the nasolabial angle is normal to prevent hyper-acuity of the columellar-labial junction.

After the TIG setback is complete, fabrication of placement of the SEG begins. By contouring the caudal edge of the SEG to reflect the desired columellar profile, and by trimming the cephalic edge to reciprocate the caudal septal contour, the SEG is fabricated to create a lock-and-key relationship to the caudal septum that permits precise end-to-end fixation of the graft (see **Fig. 9F**). Figure-of-8 sutures are placed between the caudal septum and SEG from bottom to top to create a stable end-to-end graft alignment. Further stabilization is achieved when the medial crura are then individually sutured to the caudal margin of the SEG. Unless skin closing tension is high, further stabilization of the SEG is generally unnecessary, especially when the LCT forces are also symmetrically balanced. If closing tension and/or tensioning forces are excessive, however, additional stability is required to prevent rudder-like displacement of the SEG from the midline or bowing of the dorsal L-strut. This is accomplished using cartilaginous or osseous splinting grafts in the slender nose (**Fig. 13**), or with extended spreader grafts in the wide nose or in the undersized and severely contractured nose. Alternatively, in select cases, side-to-side

fixation can also be used for effective SEG immobilization.[1–3,36] The stronger side-to-side fixation technique uses mattress sutures to secure the overlapping cartilage segments and is preferred in noses with minor deviations of the caudal septum because placement of the SEG on the side opposite the deviation results in stable midline positioning (**Fig. 14**).[36] In addition to concealing the modest caudal septal deviation, the sturdier side-to-side fixation method also obviates splinting grafts or extended spreader grafts in most cases. Graft overlap and graft thickness, however, should both be used judiciously because airway obstruction may result from impingement of the internal nasal valve. Additionally, in slender noses, airway impingement and/or visible deviation of the columella may result from side-to-side fixation when the caudal septum is located in the midline. And, as with all other structural grafts used in close proximity to the internal nasal valve, circumspect graft positioning and modest graft thickness help to prevent inadvertent nasal valve obstruction.

After placement of the SEG, which is intentionally overprojected to permit in situ refinements in graft contour, the SEG is then sequentially trimmed until the ideal position of the new TDP is established. Optimal positioning of the TDP is

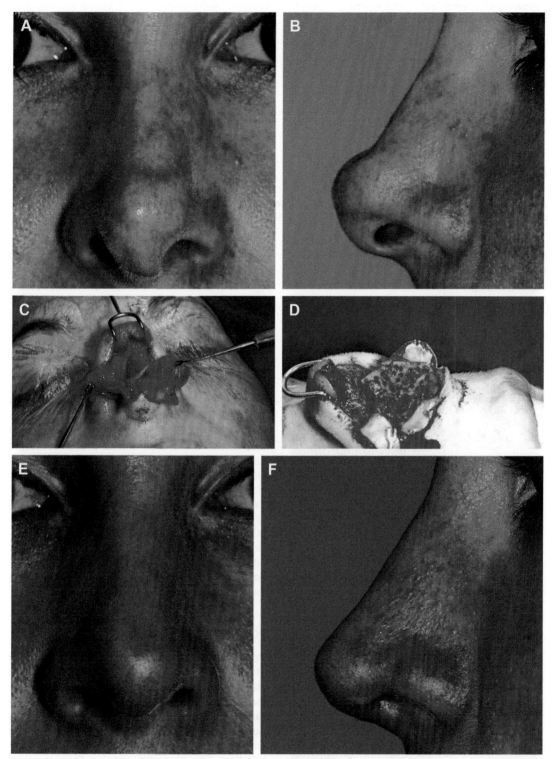

Fig. 13. Splinting of L-strut/SEG complex using perforated septal bone in the narrow nose. Preoperative frontal (*A*) and profile (*B*) views after over-resection of the nasal tip. Note twisting, foreshortening, and tip over-rotation. (*C*) Intraoperative view of deformed L-strut. (*D*) Placement of perforated (vomerine) graft for splinting of L-strut/ SEG complex. Postoperative frontal (*E*) and profile (*F*) views demonstrating improved nasal contour.

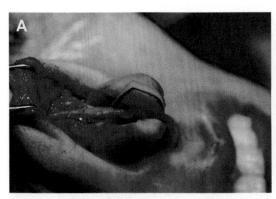
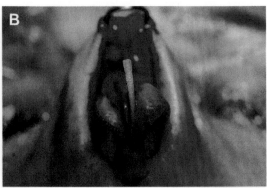

Fig. 14. Placement of SEG using overlapping (side-to-side) fixation. Intraoperative oblique (*A*) and base (*B*) views of large SEG sutured to the left caudal septum in (overlapping) side-to-side fixation technique.

determined using a quantitative comparison of the preoperative profile photograph and the corresponding computer-optimized profile simulation (**Fig. 15**). This in turn yields the approximate change in tip projection and/or dorsal

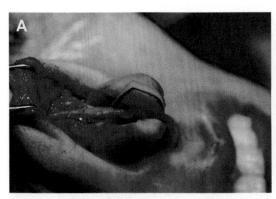

Fig. 15. Superimposed photographic comparison of preoperative profile with corresponding computer-simulated profile morph. Note measurements (in millimeters) for planned changes in nasal profile parameters.

length (relative to baseline measurements) to generate coordinates for ideal positioning of the TDP. Once the SEG is properly contoured and secured, a stable and stationary platform is then created for suspension of the reconfigured alar cartilages. When creating the new domal fold, care is taken to fold the lateral crus perpendicular to its longitudinal axis to maintain divergence of the paired TDPs and to minimize inversion of the lateral crus at its caudal margin (see **Fig. 3**E). Conversely, as each neodome is then sutured flush with the SEG, care is taken to align the suture parallel to the longitudinal axis of the lateral crus and to place the suture near the cephalic edge of the fold (see **Fig. 3**F). Finally, although some surgeons opt to forego closure of the marginal incisions when using the external rhinoplasty approach, careful closure of the marginal incision is paramount with the LCT procedure. Unless the marginal skin incisions are closed carefully and without bias, the full benefits of LCT go unrealized because enhancements in nostril size and shape will be incomplete.

POSTOPERATIVE CARE

Postoperative care begins immediately after placement of a cinch dressing followed by an aluminum splint. A circumferential wrap of 1.0-inch Coban (3M, St. Paul, Minnesota) is temporarily placed over the dorsum for temporary compression of the skin to minimize bleeding within the subcutaneous dead space during extubation. The pressure wrap is then removed immediately after extubation. An IV infusion of nicardipine hydrochloride (Chiese USA, Cary, North Carolina) is also begun at the time of bandage placement to maintain the systolic blood-pressure between 85 mm Hg and 90 mm

Hg throughout emergence and extubation to minimize ecchymosis and swelling. After extubation, the head is raised to a 45° angle and kept elevated for at least 4 weeks. A damp washcloth is then placed over the upper face, and nonlatex gloves partially filled with crushed ice are placed over the orbits and medial cheeks. Iced gloves are maintained continuously for 36 hours and changed every 45 to 60 minutes for constant cooling. Intermittent ice application is then continued for the remainder of the first week after surgery. PONV risk is minimized with a clear liquid diet, non-narcotic analgesia, and supplemental ondansetron antiemetic. Prophylactic IV antibiotics are continued overnight and oral prophylaxis is continued for 1 week postdischarge. Nasal packing is removed on the first postoperative day and sterile saline nasal irrigations are used liberally to minimize nasal crusting. The aluminum splint and outer cinch dressing are removed after approximately 7 days and bacitracin ointment is applied twice daily to the nasal vestibule for the week after bandage removal. Topical nasal steroids are initiated 2 weeks postsurgery and are continued daily until acute swelling and inflammation subside.

MINIMIZING POTENTIAL COMPLICATIONS OF LATERAL CRURAL TENSIONING
Stabilization of the Nasal Tip—Balancing Tip Forces

When performing a LCT using a SEG to suspend the modified alar cartilages, considerable tension can be generated at the point of suture fixation. Unless this tension is equally balanced, tip deviation inevitably occurs. To ensure a stable and properly aligned neotip complex, a flat, rigid, and stationary SEG/L-strut complex is paramount. When necessary, splinting grafts or extended spreader grafts fashioned from either cartilage or bone are used to straighten and strengthen the SEG/L-strut complex to maintain a straight sagittal axis and adequate longitudinal rigidity. In addition to resisting the forces of retrodisplacement generated by increased tip projection, a straight and rigid SEG/L-strut complex also serves to counter the superiorly directed forces of rotation generated by LCT. Laterally directed force vectors, however, which are also generated by sidewall tensioning, must be perfectly balanced because even a rigid SEG/L-strut complex is highly susceptible to lateral displacement from modest asymmetries in sidewall tension. To avoid tip deflection, the SEG must be pulled equally in opposite directions. Balancing the laterally directed sidewall tension of the tip complex is

analogous to a radio transmission tower that is stabilized by opposing guy-wires stretched with equal intensity. Although there is significant tension within the tip complex, balancing the lateral force components creates a steady state tip dynamic that ensures long-term stability of the central support column. Secure suture fixation of the neodomes, however, is equally important to ensure stability of the alar cartilage suspension until wound-healing processes stabilize the tip complex. This is accomplished with individual 4-0 or 5-0 polydioxone mattress sutures to suspend each dome independently from the distal SEG and augmented with transdomal polydioxone sutures to further consolidate the fixation. Although tensioning is a necessary requirement for a successful LCT procedure, sidewall tension should nevertheless be applied judiciously, because even carefully balanced forces can still destabilize the tip complex when tension is excessive. However, when the following requirements are met, a stable and symmetric tip tripod with taut nasal sidewalls is created, and long-term contour stability is generally assured if: (1) suture fixation of the neodomes is secure, (2) the SEG/L-strut complex is rigid and unyielding, and (3) the laterally directed forces created by lateral crural recruitment are applied equally.

Although achieving balanced sidewall tension is straightforward in the symmetric nasal tip, in some noses, a preexisting alar cartilage length discrepancy may cause a corresponding asymmetry in domal projection. To establish symmetric domes in the final tip construct without introducing imbalanced sidewall tension, a unilateral segmental excision of the oversized alar cartilage is required to equalize cartilage length. To optimize structural stability of the tip tripod, the author prefers to perform cartilage excision at the neodome and to avoid lateral crural or medial crural overlap techniques, which may weaken the crural span. Because the entire tip suspension is already dependent on suture fixation at the domes, this seems the most logical anatomic location for crural reattachment after vertical transection of the alar cartilage arch. Unilateral segmental dome excision is accomplished by first performing suture suspension of the smaller (normal-sized) tip cartilage and then down-sizing the oversized tip cartilage to match. After vertical transection of the oversized tip cartilage at a point 1 to 2 mm below the contralateral TDP, both medial crura are then sutured to the leading edge of the SEG. The stump of the transected lateral crus is then elevated off the vestibular skin, trimmed when necessary, folded on itself to create a lateral crural segment of the appropriate length, and then sutured to the medial crural stump/SEG complex to reconstitute the tip tripod. The end result is symmetric length of both the medial and lateral crural segments, symmetry in domal projection and rotation, and balanced tensions between the right and left lateral crura (**Fig. 16**).

Supratip Fullness

Another inadvertent consequence of an aggressive LCS is a polly beak–type profile deformity of the supratip. Because the LCS recreates each dome from a wider portion of the lateral

crus (**Fig. 17A**), the neodomal fold projects much further above the dorsal line (at its cephalic edge), producing unsightly fullness in the supratip profile (see **Fig. 17B**; **Fig. 18C–E**). Consequently, to restore the domal folds to normal length and subsequently to eliminate the unwanted supratip fullness, the elongated neodomal folds must be trimmed along their cephalic edges (see **Fig. 17C**). However, unlike the traditional cephalic trim, which resects the entire cephalic margin to produce a complete rim strip, the paradomal trim (PDT) removes only a narrow 3-mm × 7-mm strip centered around the domal fold (see

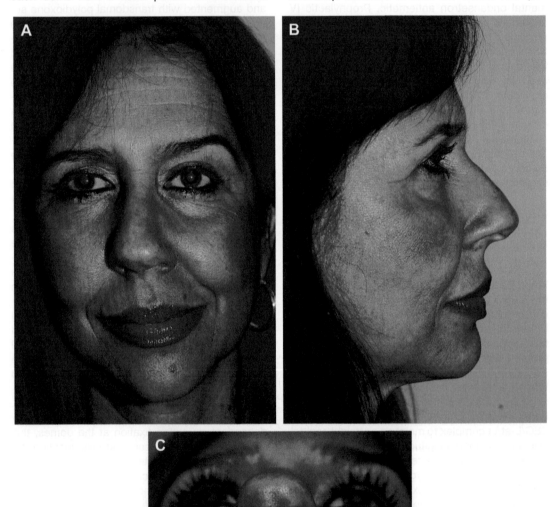

Fig. 16. Refinement of asymmetric boxy nasal tip with LCT and segmental excision of right neodome. (*A–C*) Preoperative front, profile, and base views.

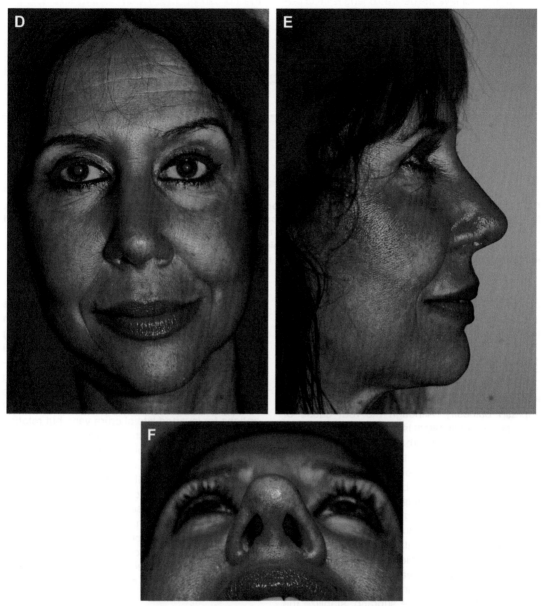

Fig. 16. (*continued*) Refinement of asymmetric boxy nasal tip with LCT and segmental excision of right neodome. (*D–E*) Corresponding postoperative views demonstrating improved tip symmetry after vertical lobular division. (*From* Davis RE. Revision of the over-resected tip/alar cartilage complex. Facial Plast Surg 2012;28(4):427–39; with permission.)

Fig. 18D, E). The trim begins medial to the nasal scroll, crosses the domal fold, and terminates on the cephalic portion of the middle crus. Care is taken to create a smooth transition from the TDP to the adjacent dorsal septum (as seen on profile view) and to achieve a final fold length of approximately 3.0 mm (see **Fig. 18**F, G). Although the PDT is primarily used to eliminate unsightly supratip fullness and thereby enhance the profile contour, the slope of the PDT and the degree of separation between the TDP and the nasal dorsum can be customized to accentuate, minimize, or eliminate the supratip break according to individual cosmetic preferences. Additionally, the PDT preserves the entire nasal scroll and, by preserving nearly the entire vertical and horizontal span of the lateral crus, structural support of the lower nasal sidewall (including the nasal scroll) is almost entirely preserved. Moreover, any slight reduction in structural support

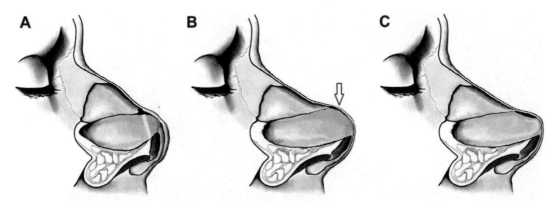

Fig. 17. Schematic illustration of the PDT. (*A*) Wide-tip cartilage with convex (bulbous) cupping of the lateral crus. Note location of natural domal fold (*orange*) and neodomal fold (*yellow*) with corresponding differences in fold height. (*B*) Appearance of right lateral crus after LCT. Note stretching and flattening of the crus and supratip profile fullness (*arrow*) resulting from increased neofold height. (*C*) Appearance of right lateral crus after PDT. Note improved supratip profile after elimination of supratip fullness with PDT.

produced by the PDT is more than offset by a substantial increase in sidewall tone generated from sidewall tensioning.

Spanning Sutures

One of the more common failures in tip surgery is inadequate treatment of supratip width and/or supratip bulbosity. Although the root cause of excessive supratip width is convexity of the lateral crura (sometimes exacerbated by excessive middle vault width), convexity and cupping of the lateral crura may persist even after an aggressive LCT. Persistent and stubborn crural convexity is most common in bulbous noses with thick and abnormally stiff tip cartilage. In this circumstance, lateral crural spanning sutures can be used to flatten and contour the lateral crura and to eliminate residual supratip width deformities after a PDT.[2,3,6] In addition to treating residual convexity of the lateral crura, spanning sutures are also used to further narrow the supratip, stabilize the tip complex, evert the lateral crura, and/or restore lateral crural symmetry after LCT. Spanning sutures may be applied unilaterally or bilaterally, as simple sutures or mattress sutures, and placed between the cut border of the LLC and either the septum, the SEG, and/or the contralateral lateral crus to sculpt the supratip to the desired contour. Care must be taken, however, to place the spanning sutures high in the middle vault to prevent unwanted constriction of the underlying internal nasal valves.

Inversion of the Lateral Crura

Another potential drawback to the LCT technique is the potential for unsightly inversion of the lateral crus. Inversion (ie, inward rotation of the lateral crus around its longitudinal axis) can result from improper placement of tip sutures, overtightening of tip sutures, excessive tensioning of the lateral crura, or combinations therein. Externally, inversion of the lateral crus results in unsightly pinching of the tip lobule with conspicuous vertical shadows separating the alar and tip lobules.[8,33,47] Treatment options for inverted lateral crura vary, but rotating (or everting) the lateral crus around its long axis using spanning sutures (placed between the medial and/or cephalic border of the lateral crus and the dorsal septum and/or SEG) often successfully lateralizes (or everts) the caudal border of the crus. Externally, proper eversion of the lateral crus creates a smooth and comparatively flat contour between the tip and alar lobules, thereby eliminating the pinched appearance. Alternatively, alar rim grafts can also be used to lateralize the caudal margin and camouflage mild pinching of the lobule.

Articulated Alar Rim Grafts

Although LCT preserves the lateral crura and increases sidewall tone to stabilize the alar rim against vertical scar retraction, poor skeletal support to the alar rim may lead to postoperative external valve collapse despite successful LCT. Postoperative collapse of the external valve is most likely to affect patients with naturally weak tip cartilage and preexisting alar rim laxity, but robust wound-healing phenomena may occasionally distort comparatively strong nostril rims. LCT may also lead to aggressive tensioning of the lateral crus with unwanted inversion of the caudal margin and subtle lobular pinching. Although a reduction in tensioning forces to eliminate

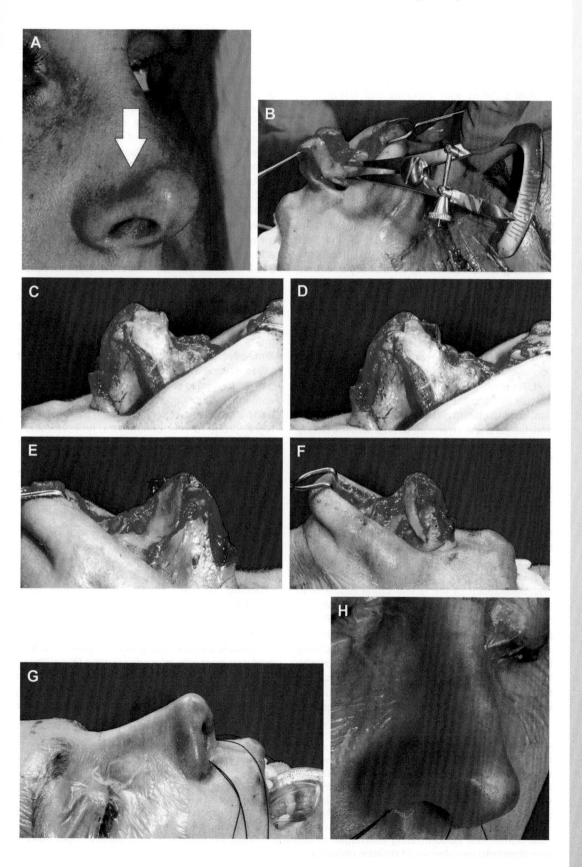

inversion is preferable, in some instances a reduction in sidewall tension proves detrimental to airway patency or supratip contour making slight lobular pinching the lesser of two evils. Moreover, in most patients with unsightly alar collapse or retraction, or in noses deemed to be at increased risk for external valve collapse or alar retraction, successful correction/prophylaxis can be achieved with small but effective alar contour grafts[48]—now commonly referred to as *alar rim grafts*. Originally described as long narrow cartilage grafts placed within a nonanatomic skin pocket dissected along the nostril rim, these floating grafts have become very effective at treating various contour disturbances of the alar rim.[48,49] The author has modified the traditional alar rim graft to increase graft stability and thus to increase effectiveness of these small and inconspicuous structural grafts. The modified alar rim graft—which the author has dubbed the *articulated alar rim graft (AARG)*—is a long and narrow batten graft, which, unlike the traditional alar rim graft, is sutured to the tip framework with multipoint fixation to enhance both contour and structural support. As such, the AARG can be used to stabilize the alar rim against primary or secondary retraction, to camouflage mild lobular pinching produced from lateral crural inversion, to augment the poorly supported alar rim against collapse, and to selectively widen the tip along its caudal-most border.[2,3] These thin, narrow, and inconspicuous grafts span the tip and alar lobules and are placed approximately 2 to 3 mm above the nostril rim. In cases of secondary alar retraction resulting from over-resection of the cephalic margin, vestibular adhesions must first be lysed to unfurl the vestibular mucosa and recreate the gap between the ULC and LLC and thus permit caudal repositioning and stabilization of the lateral crural remnant. In all cases, the AARG should be tapered laterally and beveled peripherally for camouflage. Proper positioning and secure fixation of the graft are essential because graft immobilization is critical to a favorable outcome (**Fig. 19O–R**). Medially, the graft is sutured on top of the lateral crus such that the tapered medial end is flanking (and flush with) the domal fold (see **Fig. 19O**). The graft is

also angled at approximately 90° to the sagittal midline as seen from the frontal view (see **Fig. 19Q**). Care is taken to avoid an overly acute angle between the AARG and the columella (as seen on basal view) (see **Fig. 19P**) so as to create a gentle springlike lifting effect of the alar rim. Two-point fixation—at the medial-most end of the graft and at the point of divergence from the lateral crus—is critical to resist upward displacement of the alar margin. Typically an intracutaneous skin pocket is created to house any portion of the AARG extending beyond the marginal excision. For cases of severe alar retraction, however, the pocket is dissected 1 to 2 mm further away from the nostril rim. Although the AARG may add a total lobular width increase of approximately 2 to 3 mm, this typically offsets the width reduction from crural inversion and is seldom aesthetically objectionable. When alar rim support is essential but additional width increases are undesirable, the AARGs may also be placed as underlayment grafts to negate width increases. Owing to the diminutive graft size, the economy of donor graft utilization use makes the AARG an attractive alternative to large support grafts that use large amounts of donor graft material and that may add bulk to the scroll region of the nose. In patients highly prone to scar contracture, however, additional support grafts are often necessary to prevent recurrent retraction. Nevertheless, alar rim graft/AARG placement has little downside and the author frequently uses both the traditional and the modified (articulated) graft for prophylaxis.

CASE PRESENTATION

A healthy woman presented for cosmetic rhinoplasty complaining of a large nose with a wide drooping tip. No functional complaints were elicited.

Nasal examination revealed a CTD with intermediate tip skin thickness and exceptionally weak and pliable tip cartilages (see **Fig. 19A–F**). Tip support was poor with inferiorly oriented tip cartilages and bulbous cupping of the lateral crura (in both the longitudinal and transverse planes), along with mild tip asymmetry and infratip bifidity. The

Fig. 18. PDT in over-resected nose with bilateral collapsed lateral crura. (*A*) Preoperative oblique view demonstrating supra-alar concavity (*arrow*) from lateral crural cartilage collapse. (*B*) Intraoperative view of left lateral crural remnant measuring only 4 mm wide. (*C*) Intraoperative view of left lateral crural remnant after LCT maneuver. Note cephalic protrusion of the neodomal fold. (*D*) Intraoperative left and (*E*) right profile views of overprojecting left neodomal fold marked for PDT (*blue ink*). (*F*) Right intraoperative profile view after LCT, PDT, and AARG placement. Note smooth transition from the TDP to the dorsal profile line. (*G*) Immediate postoperative right profile view demonstrating elimination of supratip fullness. (*H*) Immediate postoperative right oblique view demonstrating absence of supratip concavity.

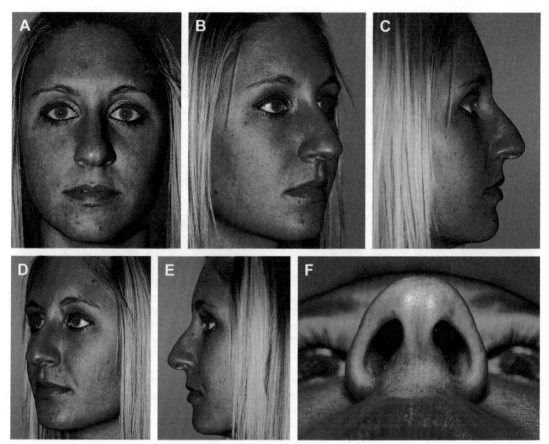

Fig. 19. Surgical refinement of the CTD using LCT, TIG setback, and AARG combined techniques. (*A–F*) Preoperative views.

dorsum was symmetric, slender, and straight, but progressive widening of the middle vault resulted from overly prominent lateral crura. On profile view, the nose appeared ptotic and slightly unprojected. Long nostrils with overly arched alar rims were present bilaterally, and the columellar-labial junction was displaced anteriorly creating fullness of the nasolabial angle. A convex dorsum with a polly beak fullness was also seen on profile view. The basal view revealed a boxy tip with columellar bifidity and thin infratip skin. Endonasal examination revealed an unremarkable nasal airway with a midline nasal septum.

Primary cosmetic rhinoplasty was performed using the open (external) rhinoplasty approach. After wide-field degloving of the skeletal framework, inspection revealed overly long, large, and convex lateral crura protruding well above the dorsal line (see **Fig. 19**G–J). The lateral crural deformity accounted for much of the dorsal convexity and for the nasal tip ptosis (see **Fig. 19**G). Round and divergent nasal domes were medially displaced resulting in foreshortened medial crura

and long, inferiorly oriented lateral crura (see **Fig. 19**G, H). The lateral crura also protruded laterally at the tip and supratip (see **Fig. 19**H–J). After dissection of the caudal septum and nasal spine, septal cartilage was harvested for graft fabrication with preservation of a sturdy residual L-strut. A TIG setback was then performed to retrodisplace the columellar-labial junction and simultaneously underproject the tip cartilages. An intentionally oversized SEG was then placed using a (left) side-to-side fixation technique for stabilization (see **Fig. 19**K–N). After component reduction of the cartilaginous and bony hump, the SEG was sequentially trimmed to the desired projection and nasal length as determined by computer-generated 2-D simulations. An LCS with 8.0-mm recruitment of both lateral crura was performed to reposition the nasal domes laterally, thereby reducing tip width and simultaneously increasing tip rotation and projection. Domal folds were created perpendicular to the long axis of the lateral crura to maintain tip divergence and then sutured flush with the SEG. Small paradomal

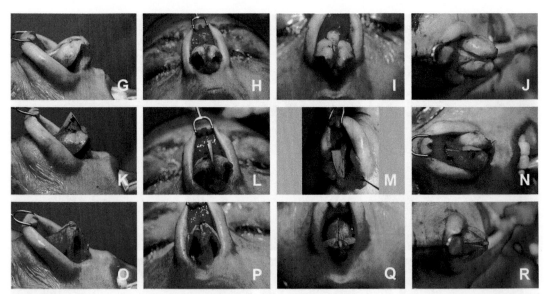

Fig. 19. (*continued*) Surgical refinement of the CTD using LCT, TIG setback, and AARG combined techniques. (*G–J*) Intraoperative views of untreated tip cartilages, (*K–N*) intraoperative views after TIG setback and SEG placement. Note difference in positioning of the columellar-labial junction before and after TIG setback. (*O–R*) Intraoperative views after TIG setback, LCT with bilateral PDT and spanning suture placement, and AARG placement.

cephalic excisions were performed bilaterally on either side of the domal fold, and spanning sutures were placed bilaterally to flatten and stabilize the lateral crura. A small augmentation graft was placed to accentuate the columellar double-break on profile view, and bilateral AARGs were then sutured to the lobule with multipoint fixation. At the conclusion of the TIG/SEG/LCS procedure, the tip complex was narrowed extensively at the supratip and more conservatively at the tip lobule (see **Fig. 19**J, N, R, and S). Tip projection and rotation were both increased, but the SEG prevented over-rotation of the tip complex (see **Fig. 19**G, O). The medial crura were also lengthened by shortening the lateral crura (see **Fig. 19**H, P) and the round and divergent domal folds were converted to angular and closely approximated TDPs (see **Fig. 19**I, Q). Postoperative photos taken at long-term follow-up reveal a natural-appearing nose with an attractive and feminine contour (see **Fig. 19**S–X). Postoperative examination also revealed good sidewall and alar rim support, a sturdy and noncompressible tip complex, and widely patent nasal passages.

SUMMARY

LCT—the combination of an aggressive LCS and a sturdy SEG (with or without TIG setback)—is a powerful and versatile technique for treating the CTD, in part because it addresses width, projection, and rotation all through a single nondestructive modification of the tip cartilage. LCT is also a radical departure from traditional excisional rhinoplasty techniques that rely on haphazard cartilage resections to achieve reductions in tip volume and shape. LCT removes little if any tip cartilage and preserves virtually all the natural skeletal support, whereas tensioning of the lateral crura, made possible through the addition of a strong and stationary SEG, serves to profoundly strengthen the lateral cartilages well beyond their baseline rigidity—a stark contrast to the flail rim strip resulting from over-resection of the cephalic margin. And because LCT increases sidewall tone and raises the threshold for internal nasal valve collapse, the nasal sidewall remains thin, lightweight, and flexible, and lateral crural augmentation grafts are generally rendered unnecessary. LCT also supplants the columellar strut graft, which lacks the stability and precision of the SEG in controlling tip position. When executed correctly, LCT fundamentally restructures the nasal tip framework by redistributing and reshaping the alar cartilage arches to produce a more attractive (and more functional) nasal tip complex. The change in skeletal architecture also creates a durable tip framework that more effectively resists deformation by the processes of wound healing. And when combined with the TIG technique, LCT readily adapts to virtually any tip morphology (including the overprojected tip) and is equally suited to both primary and secondary rhinoplasty applications.

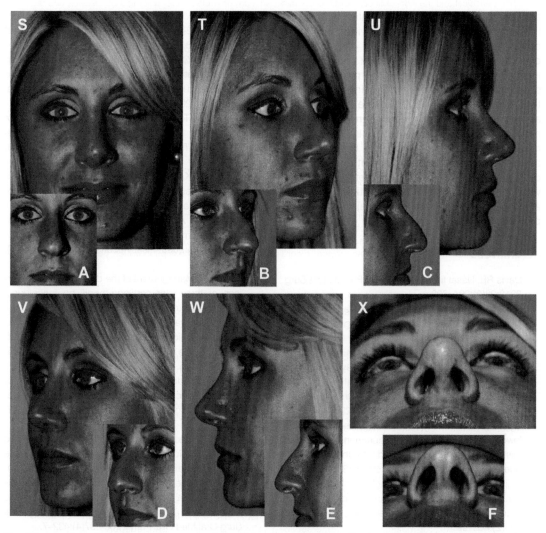

Fig. 19. (*continued*) Surgical refinement of the CTD using LCT, TIG setback, and AARG combined techniques. (*S–X*) Postoperative views demonstrating improved tip contour at long-term follow-up.

Finally, the author has been using this approach to tip refinement exclusively for well over a decade with uniformly favorable results.

As with any rhinoplasty technique, however, LCT must be applied prudently with continual reassessment of the secondary and tertiary effects of each structural modification. Proper application of the LCT technique requires prior mastery of rhinoplasty fundamentals (eg, SEG placement) and sound clinical judgment, especially with regard to positioning and contouring of the tip complex. Although LCT can create a stable and more attractive tip contour in most noses, care must be taken to avoid excessive and/or imbalanced skeletal tension because large structural loads may eventually cause destabilization and structural failure, particularly when the loads are asymmetric and skeletal

support is weak. Consequently, despite the overall versatility and efficacy of LCT, it is not a remedy for all ills. LCT alone may not be effective with extremely bulbous and rigid lateral crura because LCT is best suited to noses with weak tip cartilage and strong septal graft material. Similarly, LCT may not adequately restore extreme deficits in tip projection or nasal length especially when combined with a stiff and nondistensible skin envelope. In these situations, additional techniques may be needed to alter tip projection, contour the lower nasal sidewall, and/or reposition retracted alar rims. A graduated and stepwise approach to tip refinement, beginning with the LCT algorithm and increasing in complexity (as needed) to include ancillary techniques, such as cephalic turn-in flaps, LCSGs, Gruber-type horizontal mattress sutures,[50] lateral crural repositioning, and other techniques, will ultimately provide the best outcome for these more difficult cases. Moreover, even when LCT fails to fully correct existing tip abnormalities, it seldom precludes the successful application of adjuvant rhinoplasty techniques. Although LCT alone is not fully applicable to all noses, the wide and amorphous nasal tip with poor tip projection, inadequate tip rotation, and weak tip cartilage is particularly amenable to this treatment algorithm; and predictable, safe, and durable cosmetic refinement with satisfactory airway function can be achieved in the overwhelming majority of these patients using LCT.

REFERENCES

1. Davis RE. Nasal tip complications. Facial Plast Surg 2012;28(3):294–302.
2. Davis RE. Revision of the over-resected tip/alar cartilage complex. Facial Plast Surg 2012;28(4):427–39.
3. Davis RE. Chapter 184: revision rhinoplasty. In: Johnson JT, Rosen CA, editors. Bailey's head and neck surgery – otolaryngology, 5th edition. Philadelphia, Baltimore (MD), New York: Wolters Kluwer/Lippincott; Williams, & Wilkins; 2014. p. 2989–3052.
4. Gubisch W, Eichhorn-Sens J. Overresection of the lower lateral cartilages: a common conceptual mistake with functional and aesthetic consequences. Aesthetic Plast Surg 2009;33:6–13.
5. Sajjadian A, Rubinstein R, Naghshineh N. Current status of grafts and implants in rhinoplasty: part I. Autologous grafts. Plast Reconstr Surg 2010;125(2):40e–9e.
6. Tebbetts JB. Shaping and positioning the nasal tip without structural disruption: a new, systematic approach. Plast Reconstr Surg 1994;94:61–77.
7. Adamson PA, Litner JA, Dahiya R. The M-Arch model: a new concept of nasal tip dynamics. Arch Facial Plast Surg 2006;8(1):16–25.
8. Toriumi DM. New concepts in nasal tip contouring. Arch Facial Plast Surg 2006;8:156–85.
9. Behmand RA, Ghavami A, Guyuron B. Nasal tip suture part I: the evolution. Plast Reconstr Surg 2003;112(4):1125–9.
10. Timperley D, Stow N, Srubiski A, et al. Functional outcomes of structured nasal tip refinement. Arch Facial Plast Surg 2010;12:298–304.
11. Oliaei S, Manuel C, Protsenko D, et al. Mechanical analysis of the effects of cephalic trim on lower lateral cartilage stability. Arch Facial Plast Surg 2012;14(1):27–30.
12. Gruber RP, Zhang AY, Mohebali K. Preventing alar retraction by preservation of the lateral crus. Plast Reconstr Surg 2010;126:581–8.
13. Friedman O, Akcam T, Cook T. Reconstructive rhinoplasty: the 3-dimensional nasal tip. Arch Facial Plast Surg 2006;8:195–201.
14. Murakami CS, Barrera JE, Most SP. Preserving structural integrity of the alar cartilage in aesthetic rhinoplasty using a cephalic turn-in flap. Arch Facial Plast Surg 2009;11:126–8.
15. Keskin M, Tosun Z, Savaci N. The importance of maintaining the structural integrity of the lateral crus in tip rhinoplasty. Aesthetic Plast Surg 2009;33:803–8.
16. Kridel RW, Konior RJ, Shumrick KA, et al. Advances in nasal tip surgery: the lateral crural steal. Arch Otolaryngol Head Neck Surg 1989;115:1206–12.
17. Rohrich RJ, Adams WP. The boxy nasal tip: classification and management based on alar cartilage suturing techniques. Plast Reconstr Surg 2001;107(7):1849–63.
18. Foda HM. Management of the droopy tip: a comparison of three alar cartilage-modifying techniques. Plast Reconstr Surg 2003;112(5):1408–17.
19. Cook TA, Davis RE, Israel JM. The extended Skoog technique for repair of the unilateral cleft lip and nose deformity. Facial Plast Surg 1993;9(3):195–205.
20. Rich JS, Friedman WH, Pearlman SJ. The effects of lower lateral cartilage excision on nasal tip projection. Arch Otolaryngol Head Neck Surg 1991;117:56–9.
21. Patel JC, Fletcher JW, Singer D, et al. An anatomic and histologic analysis of the alar-facial crease and the lateral crus. Ann Plast Surg 2004;52:371–4.
22. Hatzis GP, Sherry SD, Hogan GM, et al. Observations of the marginal incision and lateral crura alar cartilage asymmetry in rhinoplasty: a fixed cadaver study. Oral Surg Oral Med Oral Pathol 2004;97(4):432–7.
23. McCollough EG, Mangat D. Systematic approach to correction of the nasal tip in rhinoplasty. Arch Otolaryngol 1981;107:12–6.
24. Alexander AJ, Shah AR, Constantinides MS. Alar retraction – etiology, treatment, and prevention. JAMA Facial Plast Surg 2013;15(4):268–74.
25. Petroff MA, McCollough EG, Hom D, et al. Nasal tip projection: quantitative changes following rhinoplasty. Arch Otolaryngol Head Neck Surg 1991;117:783–6.
26. Davis RE. Chapter 27: the thick-skinned rhinoplasty patient. In: Azizzadeh B, Murphy M, Johnson C, et al, editors. Master techniques in rhinoplasty. Philadelphia: Saunders, Elsevier Inc; 2011. p. 337–45.
27. Adams WP, Rohrich RJ, Hollier LH, et al. Anatomic basis and clinical implications for nasal tip support in open versus closed rhinoplasty. Plast Reconstr Surg 1999;103(1):255–61.
28. Byrd HS, Andochick S, Copit S, et al. Septal extension grafts: a method of controlling tip projection shape. Plast Reconstr Surg 1997;100:999–1010.

29. Kridel RW, Konior RJ. Controlled nasal tip rotation via the lateral crural overlay technique. Arch Otolaryngol Head Neck Surg 1991;117(4):411–5.

30. Foda HM, Kridel R. Lateral crural steal and lateral crural overlay: and objective evaluation. Arch Otolaryngol Head Neck Surg 1999;125(12):1365–70.

31. Gunter JP, Friedman RM. Lateral crural strut graft: techiques and clinical applications in rhinoplasty. Plast Reconstr Surg 1997;99(4):943–52.

32. Park SS, Hughley BB. Revision of the functionally devastated nasal airway. Facial Plast Surg 2012; 28(4):398–406.

33. Bared A, Rashan A, Caughlin BP, et al. Lower lateral cartilage repositioning: objective analysis using 3-dimensional imaging. JAMA Facial Plast Surg 2014;16(4):261–7.

34. Weber SM, Baker SR. Alar cartilage grafts. Clin Plast Surg 2010;37:253–64.

35. Moubayed S, Chacra ZA, Kridel RW, et al. Precise anatomical study of rhinoplasty: description of a novel method and application to the lateral crural steal. JAMA Facial Plast Surg 2014;16(1):25–30.

36. Toriumi DM. Caudal septal extension graft for correction of the retracted columella. Oper Tech Otolaryngol Head Neck Surg 1995;6:311–8.

37. Ha RY, Byrd HS. Septal extension grafts revisited: 6-year experience in controlling nasal tip projection and shape. Plast Reconstr Surg 2003;112(7):1929–35.

38. Naficy S, Baker SR. Lengthening the short nose. Arch Otolaryngol Head Neck Surg 1998;124(7):809–13.

39. Guyuron B, Varghai A. Lengthening the nose with a tongue and-groove technique. Plast Reconstr Surg 2003;111(4):1533–9.

40. Choi JY, Kang IG, Javidnia H, et al. Complications of septal extension grafts in Asian patients. JAMA Facial Plast Surg 2014;16(3):169–75.

41. Committee on Standards and Practice Parameters, Apfelbaum JL, Connis RT, et al. Practice advisory for preanesthesia evaluation: an updated report by the American Society of Anesthesiologists Task Force on Preanesthesia Evaluation. Anesthesiology 2012;116(3):522–38.

42. Feely MA, Collins CS, Daniels PR, et al. Preoperative testing before noncardiac surgery: guidelines and recommendations. Am Fam Physician 2013;87(6): 414–8.

43. Bhattarai B, Shrestha S, Singh J. Comparison of ondansetron and combination of ondansetron and dexamethasone as a prophylaxis for postoperative nausea and vomiting in adults undergoing elective laparoscopic surgery. J Emerg Trauma Shock 2011;4(2):168–72.

44. Song JW, Park EY, Lee JG, et al. The effect of combining dexamethasone with ondansetron for nausea and vomiting associated with fentanyl-based intravenous patient-controlled analgesia. Anaesthesia 2011;66(4):263–7.

45. Kridel RW, Scott BA, Foda HM. The tongue-in-groove technique in septorhinoplasty. Arch Facial Plast Surg 1999;1:246–56.

46. Davis RE. Diagnosis and surgical management of the caudal excess nasal deformity. Arch Facial Plast Surg 2005;7:124–34.

47. Toriumi DM, Checcone MA. New concepts in tip contouring. Facial Plast Surg Clin North Am 2009; 17(1):55–90.

48. Rohrich RJ, Raniere J Jr, Ha RY. The alar contour graft: correction and prevention of alar rim deformities in rhinoplasty. Plast Reconstr Surg 2002;109: 2495–505.

49. Boahene KD, Hilger PA. Alar rim grafting in rhinoplasty: indications, technique, and outcomes. Arch Facial Plast Surg 2009;11:285–9.

50. Gruber RP, Nahai F, Bogdan MA, et al. Changing the convexity and concavity of nasal cartilages and cartilage grafts with horizontal mattress suture: part II. Clinical results. Plast Reconstr Surg 2005; 115(2):595–606.

Lateral Crural Repositioning for Treatment of Cephalic Malposition

Dean M. Toriumi, MD*, Scott A. Asher, MD

KEYWORDS

- Cephalic malposition of lower lateral cartilage • Lateral crural repositioning
- Lateral crural strut grafts • Nasal tip contouring • Bulbous tip

KEY POINTS

- Indications for repositioning include deformities such as cephalic malposition, retracted alae, the pinched nasal tip, vertical asymmetries of alar base insertion, the short nose, the severely under/over projected and under/over rotated tip.
- The lateral crura of the lower lateral cartilages should be stabilized in their new positions with lateral crural strut grafts.
- Significant detail must be paid to ensure nostril symmetry after repositioning.
- Lateral wall splints should be used for 1 week to ensure proper healing.

INTRODUCTION

Repositioning of the lateral crus of the lower lateral cartilages is one of the most powerful moves in rhinoplasty. The surgeon that masters this advanced maneuver will be able to successfully correct deformities that were previously not amenable to traditional rhinoplasty techniques. Perhaps the most common indication for repositioning is to alter nasal tip contour. Deformities such as cephalically malpositioned lower lateral cartilages, retracted alae, the pinched nasal tip, and vertical asymmetries of alar base insertion can be corrected with this technique. Repositioning can also be a powerful tool to alter other parameters of the nose such as length (proportionally lengthen the lateral component of the nose to match central component lengthening), projection (enable unhindered alteration of tip projection by changing dome position), and rotation (release of the lateral crus allows complete control of the medial crura to enable fixation in any desired location). Although this powerful technique can be mastered with practice, it is imperative that the novice rhinoplasty surgeon understand the potential risks associated with the maneuver and the possible deformities introduced by improper execution.

PREOPERATIVE PLANNING AND PREPARATION

Rhinoplasty consultation should begin with a thorough history and physical examination to accurately diagnose and determine treatment-specific options for each particular patient. Preoperative photographs should be obtained in a standardized fashion (frontal, lateral, three-quarter, and base views). Newer 3-dimensional stereophotogrammetry technology provides the surgeon a powerful tool to objectively quantify shape, length, and

Division of Facial Plastic and Reconstructive Surgery, Department of Otolaryngology-Head & Neck Surgery, University of Illinois at Chicago, Chicago, IL 60612, USA
* Corresponding author.
E-mail address: dtoriumi@uic.edu

Facial Plast Surg Clin N Am 23 (2015) 55–71
http://dx.doi.org/10.1016/j.fsc.2014.09.004
1064-7406/15/$ – see front matter © 2015 Elsevier Inc. All rights reserved.

volume changes accomplished via rhinoplasty.[1–3] Digital image morphing should be considered, as it improves the surgeon's ability to communicate with their patients preoperatively on prospective changes to the nose. Function should never be compromised for aesthetics. It is imperative that the surgeon understands the patient's aesthetic preferences to prevent a dissatisfied patient, despite what the surgeon feels is an excellent result.

The surgeon should recognize nasal deformities that may not be correctable by traditional rhinoplasty grafting, suturing, or reductive techniques[4,5] and may require more powerful maneuvers such as repositioning of the lower lateral cartilages.[1,6] These may include contour abnormalities of the tip, the need to significantly lengthen the nose, disharmony between the tip and upper two-thirds of the nose requiring substantial projection/deprojection, or rotation/derotation. If repositioning is a potential maneuver, the surgeon should preoperatively pay close attention to any existing asymmetry in base insertion height, alar retraction, or notching and discuss the potential for nostril asymmetry postoperatively. The surgeon should also preoperatively inform the patient (especially the revision rhinoplasty patient) that structural grafting may be required and that an adequate supply of grafting material will be needed to change the shape of the nose and provide long-term support. This may mean the potential harvest of costal or auricular cartilage if inadequate septal cartilage is available. Such structural grafting will cause the nose to be stiffer after surgery, and it would behoove the surgeon to discuss this increased firmness with the patient so that postoperative expectations are appropriately set.

PROCEDURAL APPROACH
Overview

Before the rhinoplasty surgeon enters the operating room, he or she should spend significant time reflecting on the aesthetic effect he or she is attempting to achieve. This is especially important if one plans to alter tip contour. The ideal tip has been described by many,[7,8] but one detailed description is as follows[9]:

Frontal view

...the tip has a horizontal orientation with a shadow in the supratip area that continues into the supra-alar regions. There is a smooth transition from tip lobule to the alar lobule without a line of demarcation. The tip-defining points are seen as a horizontally oriented highlight with shadows above and below. Two horizontally oriented opposing curved lines outline the tip highlight. The lateral extent of the highlight should continue into an elevated ridge that passes in continuity with the curvilinear contour of the alar lobule.

Lateral view

...the tip projects above the dorsum with a supratip break. Most surgically untreated noses have a slightly more cephalic supratip break, preserving a rounder nasal tip. The double break is soft with a subtle shadow at the soft tissue triangle. A more refined tip is created by lowering the position of the supratip break.

Once the surgeon understands the shape he or she is trying to achieve, it then becomes important to understand the correlation between the external nasal contour and the shape of the underlying tip structures. Only then will the appropriate steps be executed during surgery to achieve the desired outcome.

Opening the Nose

Rhinoplasty can often be performed via endonasal approach, but the authors find specifically that repositioning is best executed through the external approach. Preoperative injection with 1% lidocaine with 1:100,000 epinephrine in the standard fashion should be performed before preparing and draping for optimal vasoconstriction. Rather than mindless injection into the septum, as the surgeon uses hydrostatic dissection to begin elevating the mucoperichondrial flaps he or she should be concomitantly sizing the cartilaginous versus boney components of the septum to begin formulating the amount of available cartilage here for grafting. If none exists, he or she may elect to first harvest costal or auricular cartilage, but it is often advantageous to first open the nose to determine the size, shape, and strength of grafts that will be necessary.

Standard inverted V-incision is made across the columella using a #11 blade, with anticipation of where the incision will be positioned at the end of the operation (ie, if the nose is deprojected, the incision is closer to the tip lobule; or, if the nose is to be projected, the incision should be closer to the lip) (Fig. 1). A #15 blade should be used to make bilateral marginal incisions that are then connected to the marginal extension of the columellar incision. Sharp dissection with a Converse scissor preserves the subdermal plexus to the delicate skin of the columella, tip, and soft

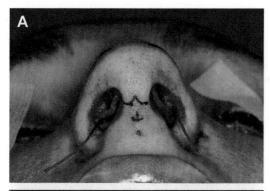

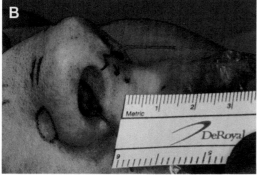

Fig. 1. Varying midcolumellar incision. Standard inverted V incision can be adjusted from the midcolumella to a position farther from or closer to the nasal tip based on plans to project or deproject the nose during rhinoplasty seen here on base (A) and three-quarter view (B).

tissue triangles. Sharp dissection may maximize vascularity and avoid excessive swelling that can be attributed to broad spreading and tearing of the tissue with blunt dissection. Three-point retraction by 1 or 2 assistants with sharp two prong hooks will aid the primary surgeon by ensuring the proper plane is maintained. Identification of the lower lateral cartilages is followed by exposure of the cartilaginous dorsum. A Joseph periosteal elevator should then be used to dissect the periosteum from the nasal bones. Most often, septoplasty should next be initiated, either by a separate Killian incision or with lateral retraction of the lower lateral cartilages and identification of the anterior septal angle. Bilateral mucoperichondrial flaps can be raised, but harvest of septal cartilage should be postponed until work on the upper third of the nose has been completed to avoid destabilization of the keystone area. Regardless of the techniques used to straighten the septum, the surgeon should ensure a strong cartilaginous L-strut exists for long-term support of the nose. The boney dorsal contour and the middle vault should next be addressed based on the desired final tip position.

Stabilizing the Nasal Base

For advanced techniques involving repositioning of the lower lateral cartilages, the authors recommend building from a stable nasal base. Attention to the midline is critical, as this is the foundation for the nasal tip. Failure to recognize and discuss facial asymmetry with the patient preoperatively can often result in the surgeon having to offer explanations for why a straight nose may still appear deviated to the patient postoperatively. Scrupulous physical examination and study of photographs can identify these and other deviations of the caudal septum, nasal spine, dentition, or lip in relation to the midline glabella. The primary surgeon should not stand in one position, but consider frequently moving around the head of the operating room table to best evaluate symmetry.

Once the surgeon feels confident the midline has been established, the next task should be to adequately stabilize the nasal base. Traditionally, options for this have included a floating columellar strut, fixed/extended columellar strut, caudal septal extension graft, or caudal septal replacement graft. If repositioning is to be considered, it is preferable to have a fixed base rather than a floating base. If the base is freely floating, the nasal tip structure can rotate and shift with the repositioning. Obviously, this will create increased stiffness in the nasal tip.

Caudal septal extension grafts can be secured to the septum in an end-to-end fashion with extended spreader grafts and slivers of cartilage or segments of 0.25-mm polydioxanone (PDS) plate perforated with a 16-gauge needle (Fig. 2). Although complex, caudal septal replacement grafts will often actually use less cartilage than attempting to straighten a severely damaged caudal portion of the L-strut.[10] Care should be taken, as this technique requires mastery in that it has the potential to simultaneously alter the tip rotation, length, and projection. Caudal septal extension or replacement grafts are the only cartilage segments in structure rhinoplasty that need to be completely straight. If the surgeon is using costal or auricular cartilage grafts, it may be wise to use any available septal cartilage for these grafts to prevent warping or deformity.

The tripod theory is a classic description to explain tip dynamics in rhinoplasty.[11,12] The nasal tip is the tabletop, with the 3 legs of the table being the left lateral crus, the right lateral crus, and the combination of the medial crura together. This theory does an excellent job of predicting rotation, projection, and length secondary to many traditional moves performed in rhinoplasty, such as cephalic trim and lateral crural steal. The theory is

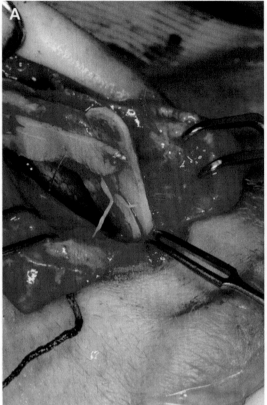
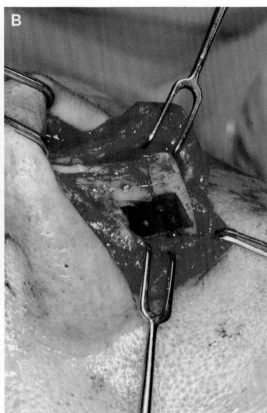

Fig. 2. Caudal septal extension grafts. Caudal septal extension grafts can be secured with bilateral extended spreader grafts and bilateral slivers of cartilage (*A*) or PDS plates (*B*) in cartilage deplete cases.

less applicable, however, if one plans to rigidly fixate the table of the tripod to the septum or septal extension graft. When this happens, the surgeon has essentially controlled for postoperative loss of projection and has controlled rotation/length. Once the confluence of the tripod is fixated, the legs are no longer floating in space, and thus can be moved, shortened, or lengthened, without fear of inadvertently altering position of the "tabletop."

The next step in stabilizing the nasal base before further tip contour work is performed is to preliminarily secure the medial crura to the septum, fixed columellar strut, septal extension graft, or septal replacement graft with a 4–0 plain gut suture on an SC-1 needle. If the surgeon is pleased with this position (see later discussion), several 5–0 PDS sutures should be used to further secure the medial and intermediate crura. Care must be taken in applying these sutures, as asymmetries can affect tip position or tip symmetry. The lateral crura should then be addressed.

Tip Contouring

The next task for the surgeon during rhinoplasty is to determine which maneuvers will attain the desired changes in tip contour and position by appropriately altering length, rotation, projection, and shape. A variety of techniques can then be used including grafting, excision, suturing, and repositioning. The focus of this review is to further discuss lateral crural repositioning.

Cephalic malposition

Perhaps one of the most common indications for lower lateral cartilage repositioning is cephalically malpositioned lower lateral cartilages (**Fig. 3**).[6] Patients with cephalic positioning of the lateral crura typically have a parentheses-shaped tip deformity[7] or bulbous nasal tip (**Fig. 4**).[13] Cephalic malposition blunts the demarcation between nasal subunits (tip/dorsum/lateral sidewall), creating excess vertical fullness in the supratip. In the more favorable orientation, the caudal margin of the lateral crus of the lower lateral cartilages, can be measured from the midline and is ideally 30° or greater. Lower lateral cartilage repositioning with lateral crural strut grafts has been shown to reliably change the orientation of the cartilages in the tip to favorably modify shape. It may also potentially reduce unwanted volume in the

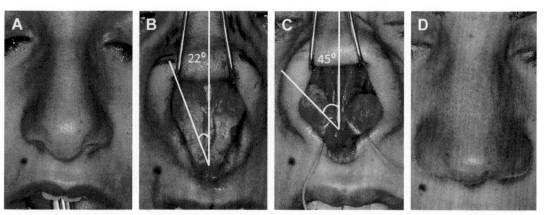

Fig. 3. Cephalic malposition. Preoperatively a wide, bulbous nasal tip with hanging tip lobule (*A*). Cephalic malposition of the lateral crura is seen with angles less than 30° from the midline (*B*). Repositioning allows increased angle between the lateral crura and the midline (*C*), seen to improve tip contour intraoperatively (*D*).

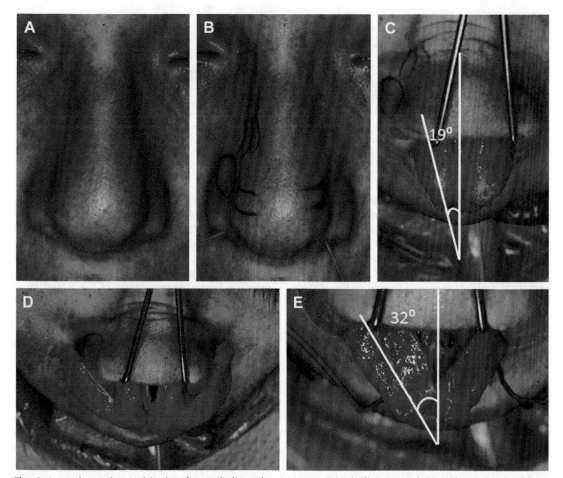

Fig. 4. Lateral crural repositioning for cephalic malposition. A wide, bulbous nasal tip with poor transition to weak alar lobules (*A*) is marked to show shadowing (*B*) before beginning the operation. Cephalic malposition of the lateral crus of the lower lateral cartilage is identified (*C*). The lateral crus of the lower lateral cartilage it is dissected free from the vestibular skin (*D*). Repositioning with lateral crural strut grafts increases the angle from the midline to improve tip contour and nasal valve function (*E*).

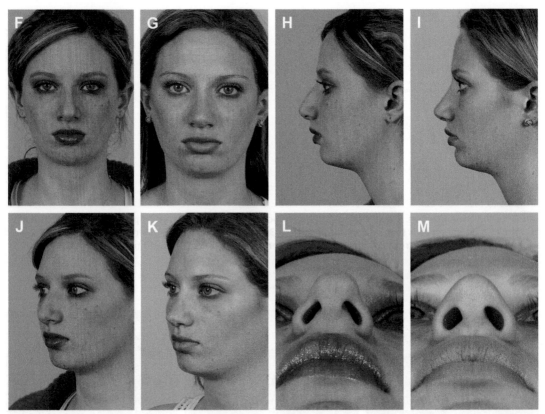

Fig. 4. (*continued*). Lateral crural repositioning for cephalic malposition. Frontal view preoperatively (*F*) and postoperatively (*G*). Right lateral view preoperatively (*H*) and postoperatively (*I*). Right three-quarter view preoperatively (*J*) and postoperatively (*K*). Base view preoperatively (*L*) and postoperatively (*M*).

supratip.[1] Repositioning with lateral crural strut grafts may also have a functional benefit over other grafts in the valve area such as alar batten grafts (Dean M. Toriumi, MD, unpublished data, 2010).

If the surgeon wishes to reposition the lateral crus of the lower lateral cartilages, the vestibular skin must first be dissected free from the under-surface of the native lateral crura (**Fig. 5**). Tears in the vestibular lining can be avoided by first hydro dissecting with 1% lidocaine with 1:100,000 epinephrine, with the bevel of the needle flat against the undersurface of the cartilage. Blunt dissection should be able to be performed if the surgeon is in the correct plane. Once the lateral crus of the lower lateral cartilages is free, the surgeon can determine what position would be ideal. Lateral crural strut grafts can be used to stabilize the dissected lateral crus and support the new desired location for the lateral crura. These cartilage grafts should most often be sized between 25 to 30 mm × 4 to 5 mm × 1 to 2 mm. The medial edge of the graft should be beveled at a 45° angle and should be advanced just short of the dome, with the cephalic margin close but

not beyond the cephalic edge of the native lateral crus. The apex of the angled end of the lateral crural strut graft should be placed along the caudal margin of the lateral crura close to but not into the dome (**Fig. 6**). This simple angulation will help elevate the caudal margin of the lateral crura to create a favorable orientation of the lateral crus. It is preferable that the graft be placed with a slight concavity facing the airway. If the lateral crural strut graft is oriented with the concave surface facing laterally it may impinge on the airway. Grafts should be sutured to the native lateral crura with the knot placed away from the vestibular skin to avoid extrusion. The grafts can also be used to flatten overly convex or concave lateral crura. The authors usually choose to also place a dome suture bilaterally to further flatten the domes and create a favorable orientation along the long axis of the cartilage.[9] The dome suture can be oriented so it is angled closer to the caudal margin medially and directed toward the cephalic margin laterally. Although it will be discussed in depth later, the surgeon must then place the lateral end of the lateral crural strut graft in a newly created pocket that

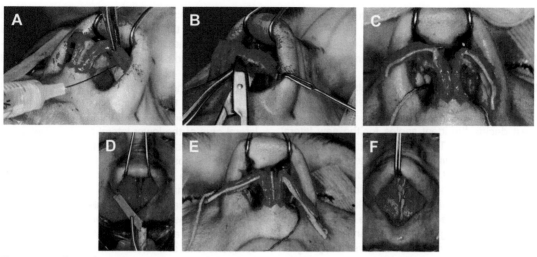

Fig. 5. Lateral crural repositioning. Hydro dissection helps avoid tearing the vestibular mucosa (*A*). Blunt dissection should be able to be performed if the surgeon is in the correct plane (*B*). Once the lateral crura are free, the surgeon can decide how they should be positioned (*C*). Lateral crural strut grafts with a 45° bevel (*D*) can be used to stabilize the lateral crura. The lateral crural strut grafts should have a slight concavity facing the airway (*E*). Domal sutures should be placed if desired before tucking the lateral ends of the grafts into their new caudally directed pockets (*F*).

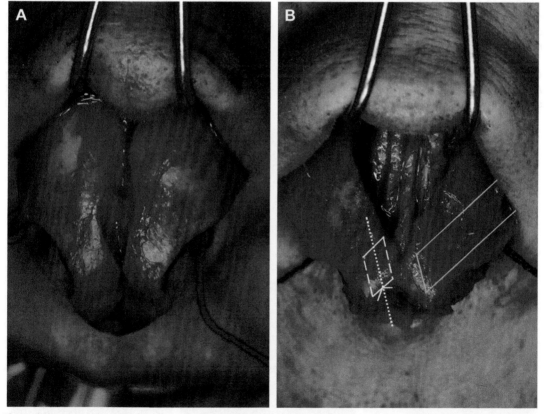

Fig. 6. Tip contouring. Cephalically malpositioned cartilages with significant convexity (*A*) are identified intraoperatively. To change tip shape (*B*) the lateral crura are repositioned caudally and flattened with lateral crural strut grafts (location outlined in *blue*). The medial edge of the lateral crural strut graft is seen beveled at a 45° angle, positioned just short of the dome. The cephalic and caudal edges of the native lateral crura should camouflage the edges of the graft. The angle (*dotted white line*) of the dome suture (horizontal mattress suture shown in *yellow*) should be oriented so it is closer to the caudal margin medially and directed toward the cephalic margin laterally.

extends toward the piriform aperture, long enough for the graft to sit without bowing.

Retracted alae and vertical asymmetries of alar base insertion

Lateral crural repositioning can also be used to correct alar retraction (**Fig. 7**) or vertical asymmetries in alar base insertion (**Fig. 8**).[14] The surgeon must decide the ideal angles for the new lateral crural positions. The pocket creation must be very precise. Beginning at the lateral end of the previously created marginal incision, the surgeon must decide the angle of dissection and degree of tissue undermining (the pocket's cephalic/caudal width). Dissecting in a more caudal fashion rather than angling out laterally can bring down a retracted nostril or can lower a vertically higher alar base insertion. If the alar base insertion needs to be corrected but the margin of the nostril needs to remain in the same location, the cephalic/caudal pocket width can be increased to prevent the soft tissue of the nostril rim from being pushed down farther. It is unusual after lateral crural repositioning to need to perform cephalic trim, as the cartilage along the cephalic margin of the lateral crura fills the space vacated by the act of repositioning.

Change in nasal length

Another indication for lateral crural repositioning is significant lengthening of the short nasal deformity.[15] This is different than the over-rotated nose, in which the nose and lip length are in good proportion to the overall length of the face, the subnasale needs to remain in the same location, and the tip of the nose simply needs repositioning caudally. In the short nose, when the central component of the nose is lengthened or moved caudally, the angle between the midline and the lateral crus of the lower lateral cartilage becomes more acute (less favorable). If the lateral components of the nose are not also brought down proportionally, the nose will have an unnatural look, often with cephalic malposition of the lower lateral cartilages, a hanging tip lobule seen on frontal view, and excess columellar show on lateral view. In shortening a long nose, often if the central component is shortened or moved cephalically, the acute angle between the lateral crura and the midline will increase (more favorable). This new orientation is usually advantageous.

Change in tip rotation

Alterations in rotation may also be indications for lateral crural repositioning depending on the pivot point of rotation. Release of the lateral crus of the lower lateral cartilages allows complete control of the position in space of the medial crus to enable fixation in any desired new location. The nose can be rotated/derotated with the pivot point being the subnasale, tip-defining point, or any point along the line between the 2. If the nasolabial

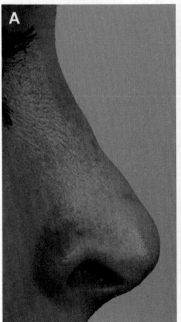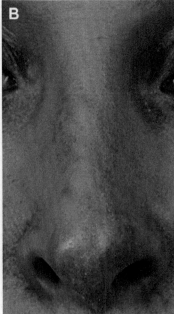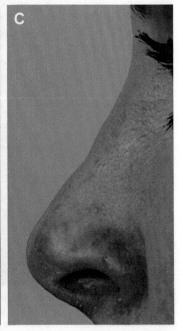

Fig. 7. Nostril analysis. It is important to analyze the shape of the nostrils from the right lateral (*A*), frontal (*B*), and left lateral (*C*) views. In this patient, both nostrils have severe retraction, but the right nostril is arched higher than the left and will require more correction.

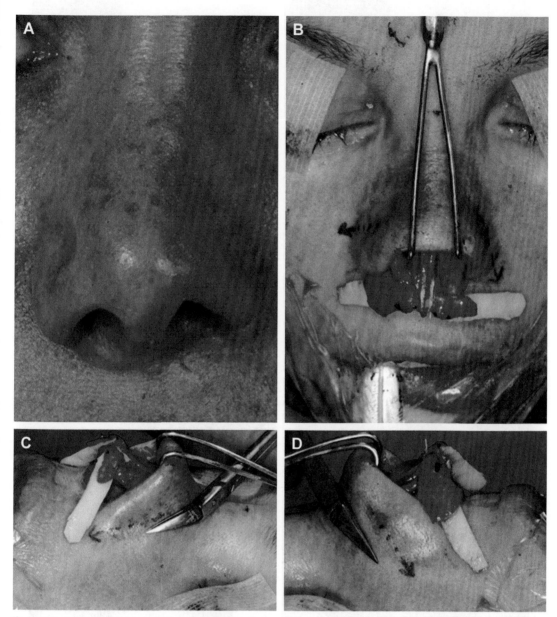

Fig. 8. Correction of base insertion asymmetry. Preoperative analysis shows left base insertion much higher than right (*A*). Correction with repositioning of the lateral crura with lateral crural strut grafts requires asymmetric pocket creation (*B*) where the left-sided tunnel is directed in a more caudal direction (*C*) compared with the right (*D*).

angle is too acute, the medial crura can be brought out anteriorly to blunt that angle (**Fig. 9**). If the nasolabial angle is too obtuse, the medial crura can be set back or moved posteriorly (**Fig. 10**). Alterations in the position of the medial crural footplates may affect the angles on frontal view of the lateral crura from the midline but often the lateral crus will need to be freed from its lateral attachments to allow this motion to take place to the degree necessary to make the appropriate changes. Although small changes in position of the medial crura can be made without releasing the lateral crura, care should be taken to watch the change in convexity of the lateral crus when the medial crural position is manipulated. Also, it is important to recognize when changing rotation that the columellar-lobular angle be controlled by the degree of infratip break, which can be independent of the nasolabial angle.

64

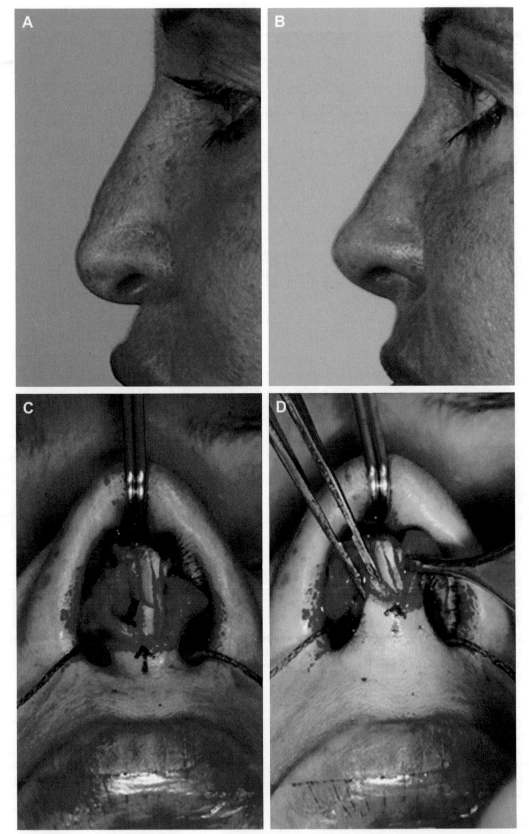

Fig. 9. Increasing nasolabial angle. Preoperative (*A*) and postoperative (*B*) photos show increase in an acute nasolabial angle by moving the medial crura from their native orientation (*C*) into a position pulled farther anteriorly (*D*).

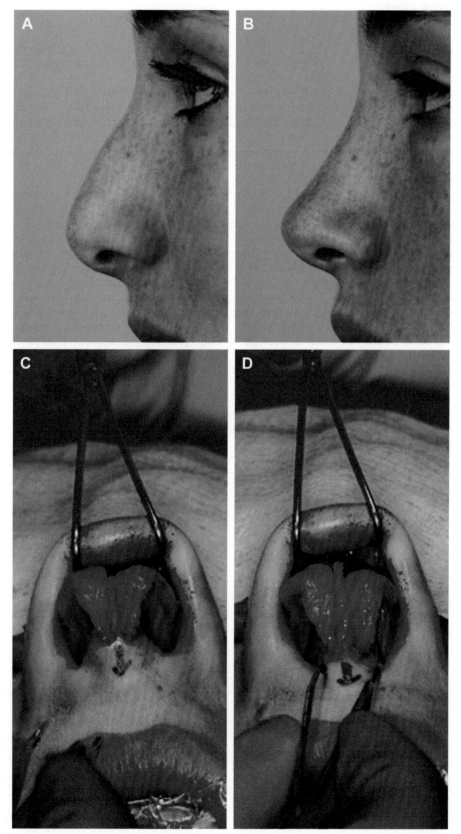

Fig. 10. Decreasing nasolabial angle. Preoperative (*A*) and postoperative (*B*) photos show decrease in an obtuse nasolabial angle by moving the medial crura from their native orientation (*C*) into a position set back farther posteriorly (*D*).

Change in tip projection

Lateral crural repositioning with lateral crural strut grafts allows the surgeon to radically change tip projection by sometimes nearly a centimeter. When freeing the vestibular mucosa/skin from the undersurface of the lateral crus, dissection is carried medial to the natural dome thereby allowing domal repositioning if desired. If projection needs to be increased, the dome can be moved laterally, similar to a lateral crural steal (**Fig. 11**). Or, if deprojection is desired, the domal position can be moved medially, similar to a medial crural steal (**Fig. 12**). The difference between this technique and the traditional techniques mentioned is that by first stabilizing the nasal base and then freeing the lateral crus of the lower lateral cartilages completely, the other variables related to the nose such as rotation and length are independent of this change in domal position. Repositioning enables unhindered alteration of tip projection by changing dome position as much as possible until the surgeon runs out of medial or lateral crus or limitations in the skin envelope. The surgeon should be aware that change in the domal

position can alter the ratio of the nostril length to tip length as seen on the base view (**Fig. 13**).

Additional considerations

If the nose is to be lengthened or the nasolabial angle is to be blunted, then the shape of the patient's smile becomes increasingly important. These changes in the nose can simultaneously alter the upper lip during the smile. Preoperative images should determine the degree to which the corners of the mouth turn up with full excursion, as this will limit the degree of change that is advisable (**Fig. 14**). If the nose is lengthened or nasolabial angle is increased by placing an extension graft that advances the columella inferiorly, as the smile goes up the lip will likely be restricted in its upward movement and a horizontal crease may form in the upper lip. Even a small amount of change can create a feeling of stiffness if not a visible crease in the upper lip; therefore, a thorough preoperative discussion with the patient is absolutely necessary.

It is imperative to appreciate the orientation of the lateral crus of the lower lateral cartilage along

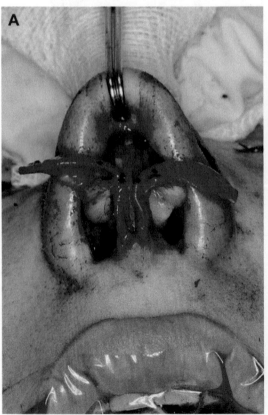 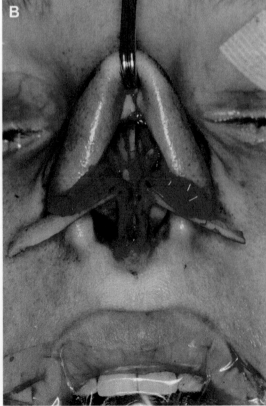

Fig. 11. Repositioning with lateral recruitment. After release of the lateral end of the lateral crus of the lower lateral cartilage (*A*), projection was increased by moving the dome position laterally (similar to a lateral crural steal) (*B*).

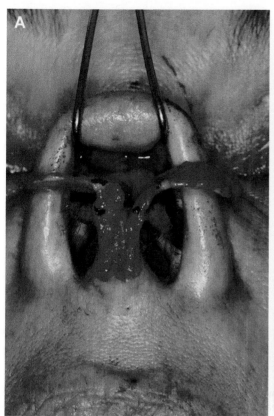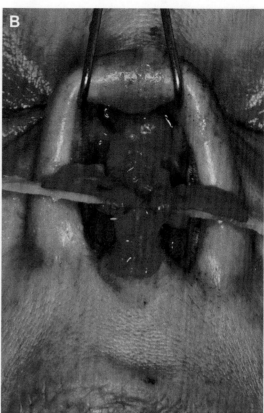

Fig. 12. Repositioning with medial recruitment. After release of the lateral end of the lateral crus of the lower lateral cartilage (*A*), projection was decreased by moving the dome position medially (similar to a medial crural steal) (*B*).

its long axis. For the most favorable tip contour, it is preferable to have the caudal margin lying close to the same level as the cephalic margin.[9] At the completion of manipulation, the caudal margin of the dome should be positioned above the cephalic margin of the dome. In this orientation, the alar margin is well supported, creating a defined horizontal ridge between the tip lobule and alar lobule. This helps prevent the pinched tip where unnatural vertical shadows disrupt the transition from tip to the ala. If repositioning and dome suturing techniques cannot attain this favorable orientation, the surgeon can still resort to using alar rim grafts to salvage the ideal tip contour (**Fig. 15**). These grafts can be placed by creating a narrow pocket just caudal to the marginal incision.[16]

Alar batten grafts can also be placed if necessary to tweak the transition from upper two-thirds to lower third of the nose. Alar battens might also be necessary to strengthen the sidewall to avoid valve collapse if significant repositioning of the lateral crus was performed. At the level of the internal valve, they can strengthen the lateral nasal wall filling the void that the lateral crus previously occupied.[17] They can also be placed to correct concavities seen on frontal view to improve symmetry in the brow tip aesthetic lines. They should be sutured into pockets created in precise locations. Care should be taken to smooth/taper the ends to avoid graft visibility.

Often, the thicker-skinned patient may need even more projection or infratip lobule augmentation, and a shield graft can be considered. Care with these grafts should always be taken to prevent visibility with contraction of the skin/soft tissue envelope over time. Lateral crural grafts or cap grafts can be used, as can perichondrium, to achieve adequate camouflage. Often in the Asian patient, the lateral crura may be small and weak and combined with thick, sebaceous skin. In these patients, it may be tempting to reposition the lateral crura, but the surgeon should be cautious to avoid accentuating a hanging alar lobule if it exists.

If, after repositioning, the surgeon wishes to slightly tweak the tip shape, he or she might consider a rectangular tip onlay graft that can be sutured horizontally across the domes. These

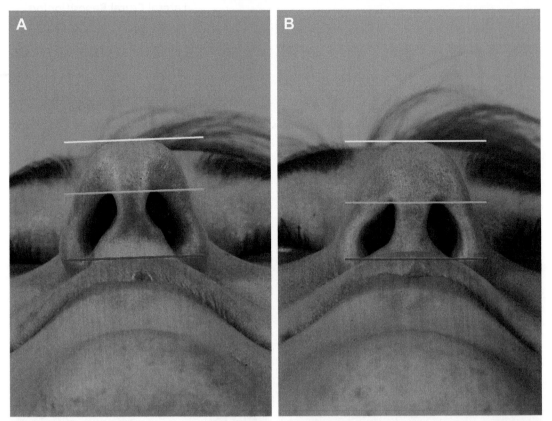

Fig. 13. Tip lobule/nostril ratio. The surgeon should be aware that lateral crural repositioning with change in the dome position laterally (to increase projection) will increase the ratio of the tip lobule length (*yellow to green*) to nostril length (*green to red*). This is seen on preoperative (*A*) and postoperative (*B*) base views.

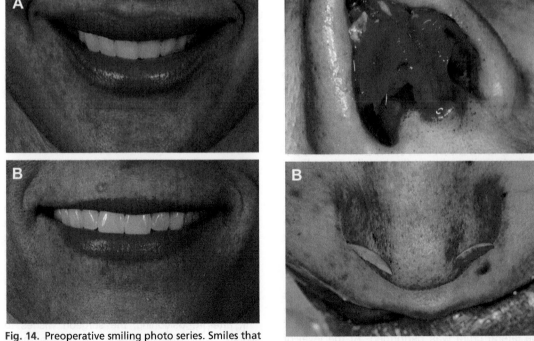

Fig. 14. Preoperative smiling photo series. Smiles that turn up at the corners of the mouth (*A*) will be able to tolerate less lengthening or increase in nasolabial angle without forming a horizontal crease in the upper lip compared with flatter smiles (*B*).

Fig. 15. Alar rim grafts. If the final position of the long axis of the lateral crus of the lower lateral cartilage is unfavorable (*A*), rim graft placement (*B*) should be considered.

grafts can be positioned higher or lower with varying widths and thicknesses to further manipulate projection, tip width, and refinement and alter the degree of supratip break. Although any type cartilage can be used for this graft, often a soft piece (cephalic trim) will function best and prevent tip bossae.

Closure

Closure should begin with a single 6–0 monocryl suture in the midline to take the tension off the skin edges and align the skin/soft tissue envelope. Interrupted 7–0 nylon vertical mattress sutures are used to close and slightly evert the inverted V columellar incision in at least 7 places. The incision should be further reapproximated with additional 6–0 fast-absorbing gut interrupted simple sutures. The marginal incisions should be closed with 5–0 chromic gut sutures in an interrupted fashion watching the nostril margin closely. If there is inadequate vestibular lining, this stitch can lead to notching, in which case a composite graft may be necessary.[14] The septum should be closed by reapproximating the mucoperichondrial flaps with a 4–0 plain gut suture in a running mattress fashion. It is critical to splint the lateral walls of the nose (Fluoroplastic septal splints, Medtronic Xomed, Jacksonville, FL) if repositioning with lateral crural strut grafts was performed (**Fig. 16**). If slight asymmetry in the nostril shape on base view is seen at the end of the operation, this same material can be constructed to form a temporary vestibular splint. The nose should be taped and a cast applied. Antibiotic ointment should be applied to all incisions and a "mustache" dressing applied to help with anterior dripping postoperatively.

Base Reductions

Often base reductions will be indicated at the end of the rhinoplasty if repositioning with lateral crural strut grafts was performed. On base view, one can see these grafts tend to slightly flare the nostrils and widen the nasal base. Base reduction can narrow the nasal base or decrease base flaring with or without decreasing the size of the nostril (depending on the location of tissue excision) (**Fig. 17**). If the surgeon is unsure whether he or she should perform a base reduction, the best answer is likely to defer reduction. The surgeon can always come

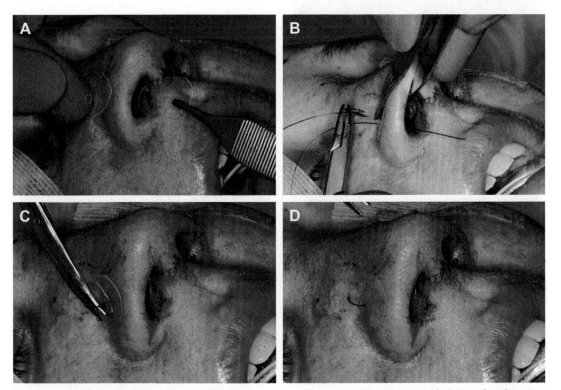

Fig. 16. Lateral wall splint placement. Radio-opaque plastic splints are sized unique to each patient for placement inside and outside of each nostril (*A*). They are sewn in place to encourage the skin, lateral crural strut grafts, and previously dissected vestibular lining to realign in the proper orientation (*B*). The knot should be loose enough to prevent necrosis but tight enough to prevent excessive sidewall thickness (*C*). Splints remain under the cast for 1 week postoperatively (*D*).

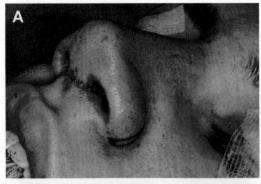

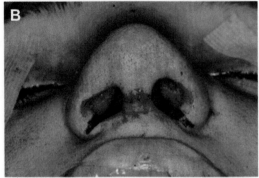

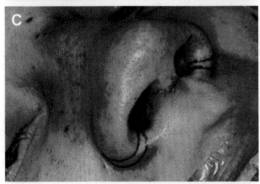

Fig. 17. Base reduction after repositioning. Base reduction can be performed on the external surface of the alae (A), internal surface of the alae (B), or full thickness of the alae (C).

back later and reduce the alar base. Typically, nostril flare will reduce over time as edema resolves and the grafts medialize. It is quite difficult to add tissue back once it has been removed. Keys to successful reduction include planning of the incision slightly adjacent to the alar/facial or alar/vestibular junction, avoiding all cautery, beveled incisions to promote eversion of the skin edges, and meticulous closure with eversion.

POTENTIAL COMPLICATIONS AND MANAGEMENT OF THEM

As with any rhinoplasty, the typical complication profile of bleeding, infection, scarring, nasal obstruction, and aesthetic deformity exists. As previously mentioned, repositioning is a complex, high-reward technique that enables the rhinoplasty surgeon to make dramatic changes to the nasal shape and function. It does, however, require mastery, and a novice performing this maneuver could potentially introduce significant deformity if executed improperly. Particular detail should be taken with this technique to achieve nostril symmetry. The ideal patient to undergo this maneuver is the patient who starts with asymmetric nostrils, as the technique will likely improve nostril symmetry if executed properly.

SUMMARY

Repositioning of the lower lateral cartilages is a powerful move for the rhinoplasty surgeon to possess in his or her armamentarium. It enables dramatic changes to tip contour and tip position as no other single move in rhinoplasty can. The surgeon should work to master this maneuver to successfully correct deformities that were previously more difficult to correct using traditional rhinoplasty techniques.

REFERENCES

1. Bared A, Rashan A, Caughlin BP, et al. Lower lateral cartilage repositioning: objective analysis using 3-dimensional imaging. JAMA Facial Plast Surg 2014;16(4):261–7.
2. Dixon TK, Caughlin BP, Munaretto N, et al. Three-dimensional evaluation of unilateral cleft rhinoplasty results. Facial Plast Surg 2013;29(2):106–15.
3. Toriumi DM, Dixon TK. Assessment of rhinoplasty techniques by overlay of before-and-after 3D images. Facial Plast Surg Clin North Am 2011;19(4): 711–23, ix.
4. Gunter JP, Landecker A, Cochran CS. Frequently used grafts in rhinoplasty: nomenclature and analysis. Plast Reconstr Surg 2006;118(1):14e–29e.
5. Toriumi DM. Structure approach in rhinoplasty. Facial Plast Surg Clin North Am 2002;10(1):1–22.
6. Gunter JP, Friedman RM. Lateral crural strut graft: technique and clinical applications in rhinoplasty. Plast Reconstr Surg 1997;99(4):943–52 [discussion: 953–5].
7. Sheen J. Aesthetic rhinoplasty. 2nd edition. St Louis (MO): CV Mosby; 1987.
8. Daniel RK. The nasal tip: anatomy and aesthetics. Plast Reconstr Surg 1992;89(2):216–24.
9. Toriumi DM. New concepts in nasal tip contouring. Arch Facial Plast Surg 2006;8(3):156–85.
10. Toriumi DM. Subtotal septal reconstruction: an update. Facial Plast Surg 2013;29(6):492–501.

11. Anderson JR. A reasoned approach to nasal base surgery. Arch Otolaryngol 1984;110(6):349–58.

12. McCollough EG. Surgery of the nasal tip. Otolaryngol Clin North Am 1987;20(4):769–84.

13. Constantian MB. The boxy nasal tip, the ball tip, and alar cartilage malposition: variations on a theme–a study in 200 consecutive primary and secondary rhinoplasty patients. Plast Reconstr Surg 2005;116(1):268–81.

14. Losquadro WD, Bared A, Toriumi DM. Correction of the retracted alar base. Facial Plast Surg 2012; 28(2):218–24.

15. Toriumi DM, Bared A. Revision of the surgically overshortened nose. Facial Plast Surg 2012;28(4): 407–16.

16. Rohrich RJ, Raniere J Jr, Ha RY. The alar contour graft: correction and prevention of alar rim deformities in rhinoplasty. Plast Reconstr Surg 2002; 109(7):2495–505 [discussion: 2506–8].

17. Toriumi DM, Josen J, Weinberger M, et al. Use of alar batten grafts for correction of nasal valve collapse. Arch Otolaryngol Head Neck Surg 1997; 123(8):802–8.

Techniques for Diced Cartilage with Deep Temporalis Fascia Graft

Jay Calvert, MD*, Edwin Kwon, MD

KEYWORDS

• Diced cartilage with deep temporalis fascia graft • Nasal dorsum • Edema

KEY POINTS

- Diced cartilage with deep temporalis fascia (DC-F) graft is a popular technique for reconstruction of the nasal dorsum.
- Cartilage can be obtained from the septum, ear, or costal cartilage when employing the DC-F technique.
- The complications seen with DC-F grafts tend to occur early in the surgeon's implementation of this technique.
- Management of the complications varies depending on the severity of the problem.

Diced cartilage with deep temporalis fascia (DC-F) graft has become a popular technique for reconstruction of the nasal dorsum. Simple in concept, the use of DC-F grafts is a choice many facial plastic surgeons make for their primary and secondary rhinoplasty operations.[1–8] This graft has been validated histologically[9–11] and has recently gained popularity because of its inherent advantageous characteristics. Its construction is autogenous in nature; it creates a reliable and manageable method of creating the dorsal aesthetic lines, and its complication rate is minimal compared with other dorsal grafts. Yet, there still exists a significant learning curve, and complications that require reoperation do occur despite DC-F's growing popularity and acceptance as a standard technique. In this article, the current techniques for utilizing DC-F grafts are discussed along with the technique-specific nuances that help to increase success rates. Complications and their management are also discussed.

Diced cartilage has been used for soft tissue reconstruction since the mid-20th century.[12–15] Peer first published on its use in cranioplasty and showed excellent long-term results.[13] Burian was also utilizing this technique for nasal reconstruction in the 1960s in Prague.[16] At that time, a curious medical student named Rollin Daniel made a visit to Burian's unit and witnessed firsthand the technique of diced cartilage for soft tissue reconstruction. Then, in 2000, Erol wrote about his experience with over 1800 primary rhinoplasty operations using diced cartilage and Surgicel (Ethicon, Somerville, NJ, USA) (DC-S) on the nasal dorsum.[17] This spurred Daniel to try the technique on 20 patients for radix grafts and dorsal on-lay grafts, but unfortunately, he did not have the success he had hoped for.

It was at this time that Daniel and Calvert began working together on a solution for the prevention of absorption of the diced cartilage grafts. They settled on deep temporalis fascia as the external wrap for the diced cartilage. Given his previous experience of 20 patients with the absorbed DC-S grafts, Daniel initially overcorrected many of his new DC-F grafts such that they needed subsequent operations to reduce the DC-F grafts. Thus, the first nuance of the technique was

Division of Plastic and Reconstructive Surgery, University of Southern California, 465 North Roxbury, Suite 1001, Beverly Hills, CA 90210, USA
* Corresponding author.
E-mail address: Drcalvert@roxburysurgery.com

Facial Plast Surg Clin N Am 23 (2015) 73–80
http://dx.doi.org/10.1016/j.fsc.2014.09.005

elucidated; given a stable dorsal base, there is no need for overcorrection when using DC-F for raising the radix, dorsal height, or defining the dorsal aesthetic lines. Daniel and Calvert went on to publish the first report of using diced cartilage and deep temporalis fascia grafts for radix and dorsal reconstruction.[18]

CURRENT TECHNIQUES

Cartilage can be obtained from the septum, ear, or costal cartilage when employing the DC-F technique. No study currently exists that shows any difference in these different types of cartilage, and the experience of the authors has been that there is no difference. The dicing of the cartilage into cubes smaller than 1 mm most likely negates any differences that might exist in the inherent cartilage properties from different sources. In fact, there have been cases in which mosaics of ear and septum, or ear and costal cartilage have been used, and there appears to be no difference in the outcome. What does, however, make a difference is is how the cartilage is diced. The cartilage must be diced into cubes smaller than 1 mm on an edge and preferably 0.5 mm on the edge (**Fig. 1**). This can be done using #11-blades, Weck blades, or more simply autoclaved stainless steel razor blades. Typically, the dicing can be done by an assistant while the primary surgeon is preparing the nose or harvesting the deep temporalis fascia, which allows for increased efficiency during the operation.

Harvesting the deep temporalis fascia can be performed though several different incisions. In women with long hair, the incision placement is more out of convenience, but effort should be made to place the incision 1 cm above and 0.5 to 1 cm posterior to the root of the helix (**Fig. 2**). However, the deep temporalis fascia can also be harvested through a temporal brow lift incision, an incision just above the root of the helix at the hairline for men who wear crew cuts, or even from a posterior helical incision with the aid of an endoscope. Regardless of the incision, the most important thing is to get a fascia graft that is large enough to use for the dorsum. This typically should be 4 cm in diameter or larger. Any smaller and there is a risk of a shortage of fascia when trying to construct the DC-F graft. Closure of the incision on the scalp is typically performed by reapproximating the superficial temporal fascia with an absorbable suture and then stapling the hair-bearing scalp skin (**Fig. 3**). Routine skin closure with sutures can be used if the pretrichal incision is used (as in a man with short hair).

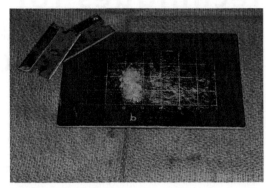

Fig. 1. Cartilage finely diced to 0.5 to 1.0 mm cubes on a metal cartilage carving board with stainless steel razor blades.

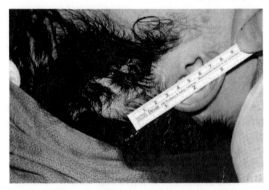

Fig. 2. Incision marking for temporalis fascia harvest in a woman. An approximately 2 cm linear incision is made. The posterior root of the helix is used as a guide to the incision. Staples can be used to retract the hair away from the incision.

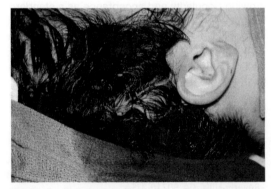

Fig. 3. The scalp incision is closed in layers. The superficial temporal fascia is closed with absorbable suture, and the scalp is closed with staples. This facilitates postoperative removal in the hair-bearing area.

Table 1
Types of operations and uses for diced cartilage and fascia grafts

Type of Operation	Function of Graft	Type of DC-F Graft
Primary rhinoplasty	Camouflage	Thin graft with 0.1–0.2 cc of diced cartilage
Primary rhinoplasty	Radix graft to raise the radix	Variable—depends on requirements for filling of the radix
Primary rhinoplasty	Define dorsal lines and smooth the dorsum	Full dorsal length (radix to septal angle) with anywhere from 0.1–1.0 cc of diced cartilage
Primary rhinoplasty	Major camouflage in the crooked nose	Full-length graft with variable amounts of diced cartilage and differential placement for volumetric balance of the dorsum
Asian rhinoplasty	Create a custom autogenous dorsum	Full-length graft with emphasis on structure for predictable healing
Secondary rhinoplasty	Camouflage of underlying grafts and structures	Thin graft with variable amounts of diced cartilage
Secondary rhinoplasty	Correct soft tissue irregularities of the dorsum from previous grafts, structural elements, damage	Full-length graft with variable amounts of diced cartilage; the greater the damage, the more cartilage should be used
Secondary rhinoplasty	Correct the over-resected dorsum	Used in concert with dorsal reconstruction grafts—either spreader grafts or dorsal onlay grafts to build up height
Infected dorsal implant	Used immediately after removal of the infected implant	Graft should be designed to replace the dorsal implant with whatever aesthetic modifications are needed for aesthetic improvement
Saddle nose deformity	After raising dorsal height with dorsal reconstruction grafts or on-lay grafts, DC-F used to create the aesthetic result	This graft needs to be placed as the aesthetic covering of the underlying reconstructed cartilaginous framework and establish dorsal aesthetic lines and contour

Once the fascia is harvested and the cartilage diced, the DC-F construct is made. It is first prudent to get an idea of what size and shape the graft needs to be in order to create the desired result. The question that must be answered is: what is the purpose of this graft? The answer can vary from augmenting the radix, raising the dorsal height, or camouflaging the multiple osteotomies of a secondary nasal fracture repair. **Table 1** outlines some of the most common uses of the DC-F graft in the primary author's (JC) practice. It is also important to get a sense of the size of the graft that is necessary when building the construct. This can be done by using dorsal sizers that are normally used in conjunction with dorsal silicone implants (**Fig. 4**). These sizers can be placed into the soft tissue envelope to determine

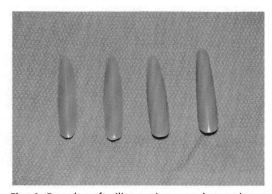

Fig. 4. Dorsal graft silicone sizers can be used as a guide in creating the DC-F construct. An appropriate sizer can be copied to build the appropriate length and volume of the DC-F graft.

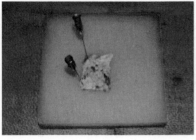
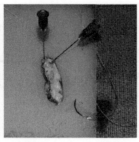
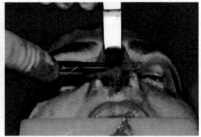

Fig. 5. The temporalis fascia can be secured with 27-gauge needles to a silicone carving block while working. Diced cartilage is placed in the center of the fascia and folded over. The lateral aspect is closed using a running 4–0 plain gut suture, and 2 guide sutures are placed at the cephalic end. An Aufricht retractor is used while guiding the needles through the radix to secure the DC-F graft into position.

if the right look is created with a specific sizer. The appropriate sizer can then be duplicated using diced cartilage and fascia.

The construct is then prepared on a silicone block with 27-gauge needles to help stabilize the fascia. The estimated amount of diced cartilage is placed into the fascia, the fascia folded over the diced cartilage, and the edges trimmed to the desired size. Typically, the width of a graft for an average dorsum is 10 mm. This takes into account the fact that the graft will shrink slightly over time, edge to edge, as it heals into position. 4–0 plain gut sutures are used to close the open edge of the fascia, and 2 4–0 plain gut sutures are then sutured to the cranial end of the graft and left with attached needles (**Figs. 5–9**). These will be used to transcutaneously fix the DC-F graft at the radix. The DC-F graft is then placed into

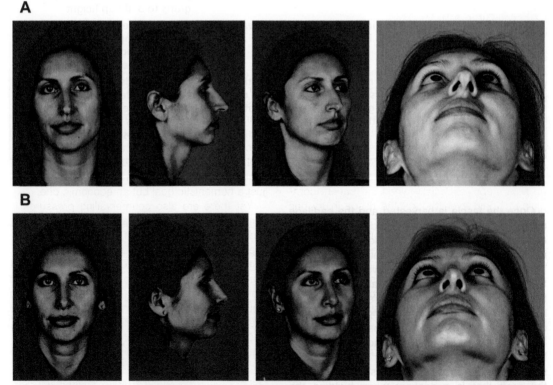

Fig. 6. (A) 28-year-old woman with septal deviation and difficulty breathing. Patient also seeking treatment for her large dorsal hump and deviated dorsal lines. (B) The patient underwent dorsal hump reduction, septoplasty, bilateral low-to-low osteotomies with addition of right medial oblique osteotomy, bilateral spreader grafts, cephalic trim, caudal septal trim, columellar strut graft, lateral crural strut grafts, alar base excision, and tip suturing. DC-F graft was used to augment the radix and the dorsum.

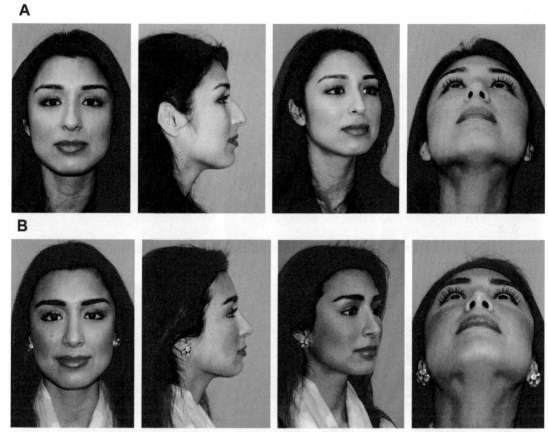

Fig. 7. (*A*) 20-year-old woman seeking primary septorhinoplasty for deviated septum, dorsal hump, and deep radix. (*B*) The patient underwent dorsal reduction, septoplasty, bilateral low-to-low osteotomies, bilateral symmetric spreader grafts, caudal septal trim, columellar strut, and tip refinement sutures. DC-F graft was placed at the radix with draping over the upper/middle vault junction. Postoperative photos at 3-year follow-up.

position with an Aufricht retractor and a needle driver with an assistant using an empty needle driver to retrieve the plain gut suture needles as they pass through the skin. These needles are cut off and the sutures taped to the forehead to secure them in place. The caudal end and lateral aspects of the graft are fixed in position under direct vision to ensure that graft position is maintained over the acute healing period using 5–0 chromic gut or vicryl sutures.

TECHNICAL POINTS
Postoperative Edema

There are many factors that determine success with this technique. The first one is that the best DC-F grafts should not be used as a major structural graft. It does contribute to structure, but only in the setting where the nose is otherwise stabilized with good anatomy and structural grafting under the DC-F. The graft size is important, because it will generally change little. What is seen intraoperatively is generally what the result will be at 1 year. The DC-F graft has a tendency to take on some additional edema at the 2- to 3-week postoperative period; however, this can be variable. The variability seems to be implicated by the skin envelope rather than the graft itself; if the skin envelope is stretched, as seen in the lengthening of a short nose, edema is less. If the skin is loose from a reduction rhinoplasty, then there will often be more edema. These issues are always better discussed with the patient before surgery rather than after.

Temporalis Fascia Harvest

The deep temporalis fascia should be harvested cleanly with as little excess soft tissue on the fascia as possible. This is achieved by carefully defining the bloodless plane between the deep and superficial fascia and also by carefully

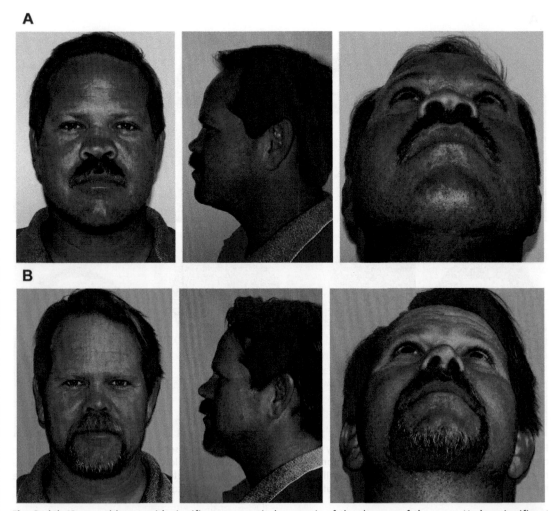

Fig. 8. (*A*) 43-year-old man with significant congenital agenesis of the dorsum of the nose. He has significant breathing difficulties and cosmetic deformity. (*B*) He underwent bone and cartilage harvest from eighth rib and composite grafts from the right ear. Extensive underlying framework was reconstructed with columellar strut, extended spreader grafts, tip graft, and bilateral base excisions. DC-F graft was used for dorsal augmentation. Postoperative photos at 7-year follow-up.

dissecting the deep temporalis fascia off the underlying temporalis muscle without fragments of muscle on the fascia. These fragments and stray tissue pieces result in more edema and scarring, which can compromise the result.

Postoperative Molding of the Graft

The DC-F grafts are substantially moldable in the early postoperative period. If the graft seems to be in the wrong position early after surgery (<3 weeks), running gloved fingers with saline on the skin can offer clues as to the graft's location and can be used to mold the graft into a more favorable position. Gentle massage is recommended in these cases, but most cases do not require any manipulation.

COMPLICATIONS

The complications seen with DC-F grafts tend to occur early in the surgeon's implementation of this technique. The learning curve is not terribly steep, but certainly exists, most surgeons becoming comfortable with the technique after 10 to 20 grafts. The surgeon new to this technique should make sure to measure the grafts they create, take a great deal of intraoperative photos (including the on-table completed rhinoplasty), and follow the grafts for a minimum of 1 year. It is also helpful to photograph the construct, the nose before placement of the graft, and the nose at completion of the case. The complications that occur are typically subtle and do not necessarily occur immediately.

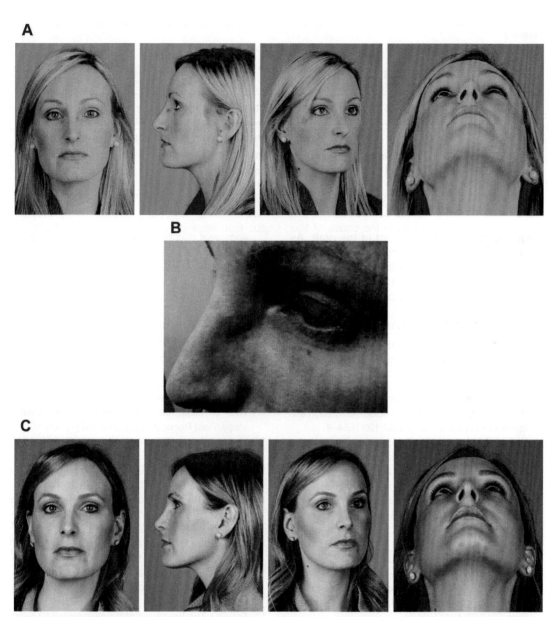

Fig. 9. (*A*) 32-year-old woman who had undergone a septorhinoplasty with alloderm complicated by wound infection 1 year later at the left medial canthal/dorsal area over the nasal bones. She was referred by her previous surgeon following negative wound cultures. (*B*) The previous wound infection near the medial canthus left the patient with compromised skin. (*C*) She underwent revision with removal of all remnants of alloderm and bone debridement. Bilateral spreader grafts and columellar struts placed. DC-F graft was placed over the dorsum to smooth the contour and provide another layer of tissue under the thinned previously infected dermis and the nasal bone.

Management of the complications varies depending on the severity of the problem (**Table 2**). If the DC-F graft becomes infected, it typically can be salvaged with antibiotics. However, it would stand to reason that the cause of graft absorption would most likely be from a low-grade infection that slowly destroys the cartilage. Thus, these complications should be followed long-

term. With malposition seen in the later period, the graft can sometimes be mobilized with a local injection of hyaluronidase that can reactivate the graft. The DC-F graft can also be removed, modified, or replaced if there are problems that are not amendable by treatment with injections or massage. Upon reoperation, the grafts are usually fairly easy to dissect, and modifications can be

Table 2
Complications and treatments of diced cartilage and fascia grafts

Complication	Number of Complications	Treatment
Infection	2	Antibiotics (oral) – 2
Malposition	5	Reoperation – 2 Injection with hyaluronidase and mobilization – 3
Overaugmentation	1	Injection with kenalog – 1
Underaugmentation	3	Reoperation – 1 Correction with filler – 2

performed from the deep aspect of the graft. As long as the surface closest to the skin is left intact, the surface will remain smooth when it is reconstructed. Typically, the graft can be replaced with transcutaneous sutures, preferable 4–0 Plain gut or for a longer hold, 4–0 PDS. The sutures can be cut at 7 to 14 days once the graft has begun to heal in place.

REFERENCES

1. Kelly MH, Bulstrode NW, Waterhouse N. Versatility of diced cartilage-fascia grafts in dorsal nasal augmentation. Plast Reconstr Surg 2007;120:1654–9.
2. Calvert JW, Brenner K. Autogenous dorsal reconstruction: maximizing the utility of diced cartilage and fascia. Semin Plast Surg 2008;22(2):110–9.
3. Daniel RK. Diced cartilage grafts in rhinoplasty surgery: current techniques and applications. Plast Reconstr Surg 2008;122(6):1883–91.
4. Gerbault O, Aiach G. Diced cartilage wrapped in deep temporal aponeurosis (DC-F): a new technique in augmentation rhinoplasty. Ann Chir Plast Esthet 2009;54(5):477–85.
5. Daniel RK, Sajadian A. Secondary rhinoplasty: management of the overresected dorsum. Facial Plast Surg 2012;28(4):417–26.
6. Savoldelli C, Kestemont P, Guevara N, et al. DC-F technique cartilage graft for nasal saddle correction. Rev Stomatol Chir Maxillofac 2012;113(2):100–3.
7. Harel M, Margulis A. Dorsal augmentation with diced cartilage enclosed with temporal fascia in secondary endonasal rhinoplasty. Aesthet Surg J 2013;33(6):809–16.
8. Tasman AJ. Advances in nasal dorsal augmentation with diced cartilage. Curr Opin Otolaryngol Head Neck Surg 2013;21(4):365–71.
9. Cakmak O, Bircan S, Buyuklu F, et al. Viability of crushed and diced cartilage grafts: a study in rabbits. Arch Facial Plast Surg 2005;7:21–6.
10. Calvert JW, Brenner K, DaCosta-Iyer M, et al. Histological analysis of human diced cartilage grafts. Plast Reconstr Surg 2006;118(1):230–6.
11. Brenner KA, McConnell MP, Evans GR, et al. Survival of diced cartilage grafts: an experimental study. Plast Reconstr Surg 2006;117(1):105–15.
12. Young F. Autogenous cartilage grafts. Surgery 1941;10:7.
13. Peer LA. Diced cartilage grafts. Arch Otolaryngol 1943;38:156–65.
14. Peer LA. Reconstruction of the auricle with diced cartilage grafts in a Vitallium ear mold. Plast Reconstr Surg 1948;3:653–66.
15. Wilflingseder P. Cranioplasties by means of diced cartilage and split rib grafts. Minerva Chir 1983;38:837–43.
16. Burian K. Rhinosurgical interventions in the hypophysical region. Arch Otorhinolaryngol 1974;207(2):401–8.
17. Erol OO. The Turkish delight: a pliable graft for rhinoplasty. Plast Reconstr Surg 2000;105(6):2229–41 [discussion: 2242–3].
18. Daniel RK, Calvert JW. Diced cartilage grafts in rhinoplasty surgery. Plast Reconstr Surg 2004;113(7):2156–71.

Contemporary Techniques for Effective Nasal Lengthening

Kristopher Katira, MD[a], Bahman Guyuron, MD[b],*

KEYWORDS

- Rhinoplasty • Revision rhinoplasty • Secondary rhinoplasty • Short nose • Nasal lengthening
- Tongue-and-groove technique • Septal extension graft • Columellar strut

KEY POINTS

- The correct lengthening procedure is one that elongates deficient/deformed structures and respects overall nasal and facial aesthetic proportions.
- More significant length deficiency requires elongation of the dorsal frame with septal extension grafts, composite grafts, or the tongue-and-groove technique.
- A tongue-and-groove construct consists of paired septal extension spreader grafts that interdigitate with a columellar strut.
- Lateral crural repositioning, alar rim grafting, lateral crural strut grafting, composite grafting, or V-Y mucosal advancements may be necessary if lateral tissues do not advance with central components.
- It may be prudent to sacrifice some central lengthening if there are soft tissue limitations preventing concurrent advancement of lateral tissues.

 Videos of the tongue-and-groove technique accompany this article at http://www.facialplastic. theclinics.com/

INTRODUCTION OR OVERVIEW

The short nose represents one of the most challenging problems in rhinoplasty. The shorter the nose, the greater the challenge. A mastery of nasofacial analysis and rhinoplasty dynamics as well as a thorough understanding of the cause of the shortening are prerequisites to designing effective nasal lengthening procedures.

Nasal length is typically measured from radix to pronasale, and, in an otherwise idealized face, nasal length should equal two-thirds the height of the midface (supraorbitale to subnasale) or the distance from stomion to menton. As an alternative, the Goode ratio defines the ideal nasal length as a ratio with respect to nasal projection (5:3).[1–6] Although nasal length can be strictly defined in this manner, the short nose deformity often presents as a constellation of features. Hallmark features of the short nose include decreased nasal bridge length, increased nostril show, retracted alae, cephalic tip over-rotation, a low or deep radix, and a long upper lip.[7,8] Given the variety of characteristics that comprise this deformity, certain investigators have advocated algorithmic classification systems to help guide operative approaches.[9]

Disclosure: The authors have nothing to disclose related to the content of this article.
[a] Department of Plastic Surgery, University Hospitals Case Medical Center, 11100 Euclid Avenue, Cleveland, OH 44106, USA; [b] Department of Plastic Surgery, University Hospitals Case Medical Center, 29017 Cedar Road, Cleveland, OH 44124, USA
* Corresponding author.
E-mail address: bahman.guyuron@uhhospitals.org

facialplastic.theclinics.com

The short nose can be further understood in terms of cause. Deformities are classified as either acquired or congenital, with most cases being acquired. In the past, the most common cause was iatrogenic, characterized by cephalic over-rotation. Additional causes of acquired deformities include trauma, cocaine insufflation, autoimmune disorders, local or systemic infections, or a history of oncologic nasal surgery.[10,11] In acquired cases, scarred or contracted tissues, fractured skeletal structures, or loss of graft sites can be encountered. Among congenital causes, short noses can arise from uniform hypoplasia of nasal anatomic structures, such as the nasal spine.

As expected for a deformity with diverse features and causes, many different lengthening techniques have been described, including craniofacial osteotomies, locoregional flaps, cartilage grafts, and incisional/dissection techniques. Regardless of the choice of technique or approach, effective nasal lengthening procedures are typically accomplished using well-accepted principles. Principles of nasal lengthening include (1) precise assessment of length deficiency; (2) accurate identification of deficient tissues; (3) adequate release of the soft tissue envelope; and (4) pertinent modification of deficient skin, mucosa, and/or skeletal deformities to restore length.

In the experience of the senior author (BG), the tongue-and-groove technique is a versatile means of achieving consistent, precise, and stable nasal lengthening in most patients with moderate to severe shortening. This technique uses a custom construct consisting of paired septal extension spreader grafts that interdigitate with a columellar strut. Ancillary techniques, such as alar or lateral crural modifications, soft tissue undermining, mucosal advancement flaps, or interpositional composite grafting may be indicated in specific circumstances. In cases of mild anterior shortening, tip grafting in the form of shield grafts may be preferred.

TREATMENT GOALS AND PLANNED OUTCOMES

The ultimate goal is to appropriately lengthen deficient tissues, restoring facial harmony and preserves nasal function. In order to accomplish this goal, the surgeon must understand the cause of nasal shortening, identify specific anatomic structures that are deficient, and execute a sound operative plan in a safe and practical manner. Many of the lengthening techniques, especially in cases of severe shortening, are associated with either unstable alignment or significant rigidity. The ideal lengthening technique is one that offers versatility

in elongation and optimizes the suppleness of the nasal base and stability of the nasal construct.

PREOPERATIVE PLANNING AND PREPARATION

Standard aspects of the preoperative rhinoplasty evaluation apply in cases of short noses. Inquiry about previous nasal surgery, trauma, or substance abuse is particularly important. If prior radiographic imaging was obtained, these studies should be reviewed. If the patient had previous surgery, assessment of donor sites is essential. An understanding of patient expectations is also important, because it is crucial for the surgeon to consider the patient's exact wishes. A review of factors contributing to excessive bleeding can also be performed, including a history of procedural bleeding, known or suspected coagulopathy, and a review of pharmaceutical agents commonly associated with increased bleeding.[12] A comprehensive questionnaire can be helpful in the assessment of nasal dysfunction, including an assessment of breathing dynamics, rhinitis, or sinusitis. Questions related to a history of headache or migraines can guide specific rewarding ancillary procedural interventions. For instance, rhinogenic migraine headaches start from behind the eyes, with headaches arising at night or with atmospheric pressure changes. In patients with severe headache symptoms that do not respond to conventional medical therapies, septorhinoplasty or endoscopic nasal surgery may be indicated to address disorders such as septal spurs or contact points, septum bullosa, and concha bullosa.[13–15]

After a thorough history is obtained, standardized nasofacial analysis is performed to identify nasal flaws and sources of facial disharmony. Observation of patient skin thickness allows an understanding of the way that osseocartilaginous modifications manifest after skin redraping. The ideal radix is 4 mm deep in men and 6 mm deep in women. Women should have a well-defined supratip break. The nasolabial angle for men is 94° to 97° and 97° to 100° for women.[16,17] The columella protrudes 3 to 4 mm caudal to the alar rim in optimally positioned alae. The septum is observed internally for deviation. A drafting film is placed over profile and anteroposterior (AP) views of life-sized photographs and marked systematically to define flaws in the nasofrontal groove, dorsum, tip, alar bases, and chin position, using the cephalometric analysis described by the senior author (Guyuron[18]). A prefabricated template is also used to create an ideal nasal outline in a segmental fashion.

With the general patient assessment complete, a refined understanding of the details of nasal shortening should be sought. With regard to nasal length assessment, it is crucial to distinguish between isolated anterior and pan-nose shortening and to consider the anatomic implications of these observations. Anterior shortening is suggested by isolated tip over-rotation or lobule deficiency, whereas pan-nose shortening represents total length deficiency. Anterior shortening can arise from over-resection of the anterocaudal septum, collapse of the septum from a caudal blow to the nose, or chemical septal destruction as with cocaine. In these cases, the columella and nasal spine may be adequately positioned. In contrast, pan-nose shortening is a combination of anterior and posterior shortening, as seen in some congenital cases.

An assessment of the alae and the quality of the soft tissues is also essential, because they can thwart efforts to achieve a uniform nasal lengthening. Actual or potential alar retraction, if not accounted for preoperatively, can compromise the aesthetic result or limit the amount of central tissue advancement. Likewise, soft tissue contracture along mucosal or external tissues can resist lengthening. In cases of severe contracture, structures such as the columella may not be supple enough to be displaced caudally if soft tissues are not widely released.[19]

Determinations of cartilage availability and priority are especially important in cases of previous nasal trauma or in cases of secondary rhinoplasty. Septal cartilage may not be available, and conchal or costal cartilage may have been used previously. Understanding this point allows the surgeon to prioritize grafts based on limited donor cartilage availability. Depending on the specific lengthening procedure, the availability of strong, straight pieces of cartilage for the dorsum and columellar strut are a top priority; followed by spreader grafts, tip grafts, alar rim grafts, radix grafts, and nasal spine grafts, in order of decreasing priority.[20]

PATIENT POSITIONING/PREPARATION

Patients are typically placed in the supine position. The head is placed on a horseshoe head support and as close to the edge of the operating room table as possible. Both arms are tucked. The face and the anterior chest wall are prepped. Life-sized photographs can be taped on an intravenous pole and placed nearby for intraoperative review. Once general anesthesia is induced, the patient is intubated using an oral ray endotracheal tube.

Injection of local anesthesia is performed in the following manner. To minimize the systemic effects of epinephrine, such as tachyarrhythmia and hypertension, staged injections with increasing concentrations of epinephrine are performed. Xylocaine containing 1:200,000 epinephrine is used first. In cases of planned turbinectomy, turbinates are injected. Gauze packing soaked in oxymetazoline hydrochloride or phenylephrine is then placed as far posteriorly and cephalically as possible. The radix is then injected, followed by soft tissues along the lateral and medial surfaces of the nasal bones. The dorsal septum on either side of the nasal roof is then injected, followed by the lining of the vomer and the floor of the nose as far posteriorly and caudally as possible. After waiting several minutes for the epinephrine to work, the same steps are followed with 0.5% ropivacaine containing 1:100,000 epinephrine. This double-injection method ensures maximal vasoconstriction, limits postoperative narcotic use, and provides an opportunity for intraoperative visibility.

PROCEDURAL APPROACH

Choice of operative approach and technique ultimately depends on the type and severity of length deficiency. If there is mild anterior deficiency in the infratip lobule or columella, a shield-tip graft can be used. In contrast, if there is moderate to severe shortening, then the dorsal nasal framework must be elongated. Elongation of the dorsum can be accomplished using septal extension grafts, composite grafts in case of severe lining deficiency, or the tongue-and-groove technique. In addition, ancillary maneuvers can be performed to ensure adequate lengthening and balanced proportions, including soft tissue undermining, upper lateral cartilage derotation, lateral crural grafting or alar grafting, and tip suturing.

SHIELD-TIP GRAFT

Mild shortening attributed to the infratip lobule or anterior columella can be corrected using a shield-type tip graft. **Fig. 1** shows an example of a patient who would benefit from this technique. If the only modification required is a shield-type tip graft, this can be placed endonasally through a marginal incision extending laterally from the anterior portion of the columella. However, in most cases of shortening, other flaws are present, such as alar retraction, which requires additional modifications.

In all cases except for minor tip graft modifications, an external rhinoplasty approach is preferred. A transcolumellar incision is marked in the narrowest portion of the columella using double-hook retraction to pull the domes

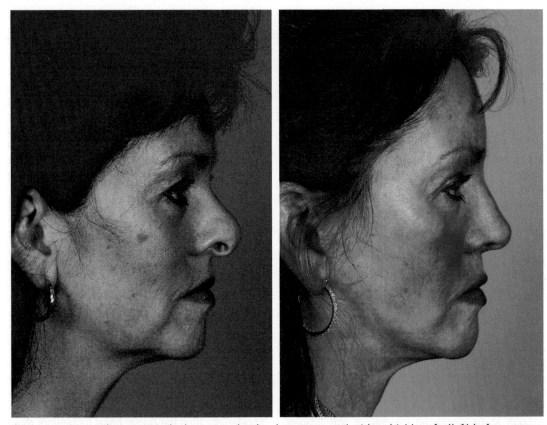

Fig. 1. A patient with an anteriorly short nose that has been corrected with a shield graft: (*left*) before surgery, (*right*) after surgery. (*From* Guyuron B. Elongation of the short nose. In: Guyuron B, editor. Rhinoplasty. New York: Elsevier; 2012. p. 183; with permission.)

anteriorly. The stair-step transcolumellar incision is connected to bilateral marginal incisions along the caudal edge of the medial and lateral crura. This incision provides the least visible scar and the best alignment of the wound margins. Modifications of operative approach may be required in cases of traumatic lacerations.

After exposure of the lower lateral cartilages, the medial crura are approximated. A shield graft is carved using a tip punch device.[21] Septal cartilage is preferred but conchal cartilage can be used when there is a paucity of donor septum. The punch creates an anatomic graft with 2 round cephalic segments and an infratip portion, which emulate the shape of the natural domes and infratip (**Fig. 2**). A second layer can be applied depending on the amount of elongation needed and the thickness of the first graft. Only a single graft is usually required.

This shield-tip graft can be used in 2 different ways, depending on whether tip projection deficiency coexists. If projection is needed, the graft can be draped over the existing domes. If projection is not needed, the shield graft can be added caudal to the domes to achieve lengthening only.

The margins of the graft are beveled, especially in patients with thin skin, to minimize graft visibility. The graft is sewn in position in a precise three-dimensional manner once adequately positioned (**Fig. 3**), and 6-0 polyglactin is used because it ties easily and the soft ends typically do not create contour irregularities.

In these patients, actual or potential alar retraction can be corrected using either alar rim grafts or a mucosal V-Y advancement. These techniques can advance the ala caudally and restore congruity between the alae and the lobule.[22,23]

TONGUE-AND-GROOVE TECHNIQUE

In cases of moderate to severe length deficiency, options for elongation include septal extension grafts, composite grafts, or a tongue-and-groove construct. Although septal extension grafts can provide the intended lengthening, they are prone to malposition over time; they can shift or rotate because they are not stably fixed to the septum on both sides. Furthermore, those extension grafts that are fixed to one side of the septum are not exactly anatomic and may shift the tip to side to

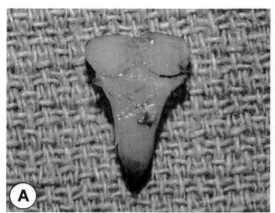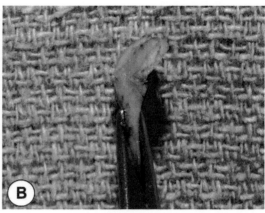

Fig. 2. A shield graft is harvested using a tip punch: front view (*A*), profile view (*B*). (*From* Guyuron B. Elongation of the short nose. In: Guyuron B, editor. Rhinoplasty. New York: Elsevier; 2012. p. 181; with permission.)

which the extension graft is sutured. A tongue-and-groove construct circumvents these problems by reinforcing paired septal extended spreader grafts with a columellar strut. This tongue-and-groove framework allows a more stable, long-lasting construct and gives the surgeon control of the amount of nasal elongation. This stability, durability, and versatility make the tongue-and-groove technique an optimal choice for correction of moderate to severe deformities.

The tongue-and-groove technique begins with an external approach. If indicated, the dorsum is refined and osteotomies are completed. Two long spreader grafts are then harvested, ideally from the septum. Rib is an acceptable donor, whereas conchal cartilage is not. These spreader grafts extend from the nasal bones to beyond the anterocaudal septum in proportion to the amount of lengthening desired (**Fig. 4**A, B). For instance, if the nose requires 4 mm of lengthening, the spreader grafts extend beyond the septum by

4 mm. Grafts are sewn into position using 2 or 3 double-armed 5-0 polyglactin sutures (see **Fig. 4**C–E); 5-0 polydioxanone (PDS) is used to suture the upper lateral cartilages to the septum, which in turn provides longer stability for the extended spreader grafts.

The next step is to design a columellar strut that interdigitates with the spreader grafts to provide the desired amount of lengthening. The shape and dimensions of the strut depend on the amount of projection and lengthening desired. For instance, if the anterior nasal spine and caudal septum are in proper position, a triangular-shaped strut is fashioned. If the posterior columella needs to be advanced, a rectangular-shaped strut is designed. Regardless of shape, the dimensions of the strut depend on the width of the medial crura and the amount of lengthening desired. For instance, if the medial crura are 4 mm wide and 4 mm of lengthening is necessary, then the cephalocaudal dimension of the strut would be 8 mm. If the columellar strut is designed to

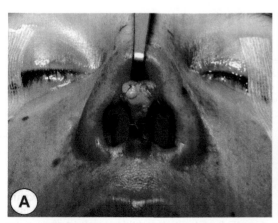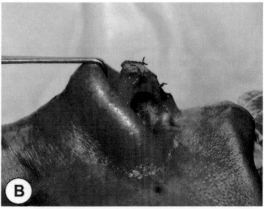

Fig. 3. The shield graft is sutured in position three-dimensionally: basilar view (*A*), profile view (*B*). (*From* Guyuron B. Elongation of the short nose. In: Guyuron B, editor. Rhinoplasty. New York: Elsevier; 2012. p. 182; with permission.)

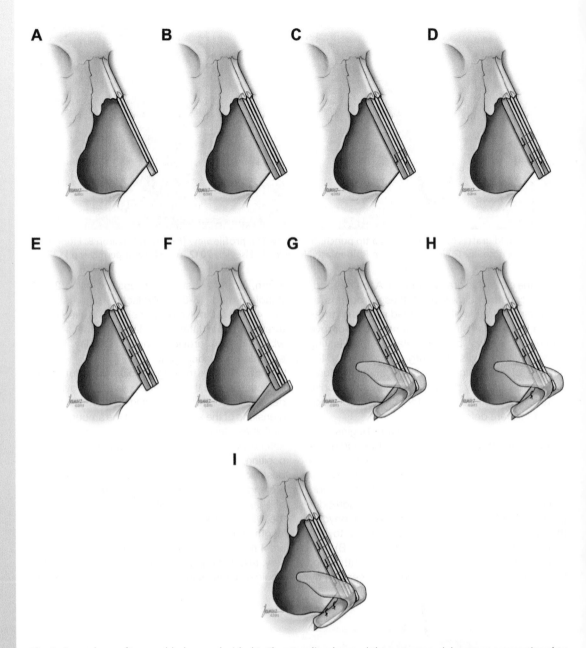

Fig. 4. Spreader grafts are added on each side (*A, B*), extending beyond the anterocaudal septum proportional to the elongation necessary and fixed to the septum using 3 mattress sutures of 5-0 PDS (*C–E*). A columellar strut is placed in a position that has an AP width equal to the required elongation of the nose plus the width of the medial crura (*F*). The medial crura are sutured to the newly placed strut in at least 2 places (*G–I*). PDS, polydioxanone. (*From* Guyuron B. Elongation of the short nose. In: Guyuron B, editor. Rhinoplasty. New York: Elsevier; 2012. p. 184–5; with permission.)

be triangular and the footplates of the medial crura are divergent, the clinician must consider how far the columella and the subnasale will be advanced when the medial crura are approximated. A groove is created in the nasal spine to accommodate the posterior end of the columellar strut and the strut is inserted in this ~~this~~ groove first. Should there be

any potential for dislodgement of the columellar strut, it is fixed to the anterior nasal spine periosteum with a 5-0 PDS suture. The strut is then sutured to the medial crura in at least 2 sites with 5-0 PDS (see **Fig. 4F–I**). Video 1 shows this sequence.[24]

The columellar strut interfaces with the extended spreader grafts and the medial crura in a precise manner. First, the columellar strut should not extend beyond the dorsum, except for the portion between the medial crura. Second, the portion of strut between the medial crura should extend only 6 to 8 mm beyond the dorsum cephalically, depending on the thickness of the skin, and the strut should not extend beyond the most projected portion of the domes. Third, the portion of the strut that extends anterior to the spreader grafts between the medial crura should not be wider than the medial crura. This configuration collectively guarantees precise lengthening as well as avoidance of contour and supratip deformities. Unless increased tip projection is required, the columella strut is not sutured to the extended spreader grafts or the septum. Suturing contributes to nasal rigidity, which is not ideal. If additional projection is needed, 5-0 clear nylon is used to suture the strut to the medial crura in a more projected position.

Once central lengthening has been accomplished with a tongue-and-groove construct, the next step is to ensure that the lateral structures and the external soft tissues will advance. The lateral crura are exposed, completely mobilized, and rotated caudally into a new soft tissue pocket. A Gunter-type lateral crural strut graft may be useful to strengthen external valves or improve the appearance of the alae. Patients with contracted soft tissues often require wide release with elevation of soft tissues cephalically along the dorsum and nasal bones. If soft tissue release is not possible, a mucosal incision is made and an elliptical composite conchal cartilage and skin graft is applied cephalad to the lower lateral cartilages and extended to the membranous septum. However, this is seldom necessary.

For patients in whom central lengthening cannot be accomplished without significant alar retraction, a compromise often has to be made. If lateral tissue retraction would persist despite corrective maneuvers, it is more prudent to sacrifice some central lengthening at the expense of balancing lateral nasal elements. The same caution needs to be exercised in the case of significant skin shortage when the columellar repair seems too tight. Attempts should be directed at further undermining the cephalic soft tissues. However, if this fails to yield enough soft tissue freedom for a comfortable repair, the compromise should be on the side of a slightly shorter nose rather than having necrosis of the columellar skin, which is extremely difficult to reconstruct.

After ancillary maneuvers and closure are performed, Doyle stents and a nasal splint are applied in the following manner. Mastisol® and 12-mm (0.5 inch) Steri-Strips™ are applied before application of a splint. A combination metal and Aquaplast™ splint is applied and taped in position with Steri-Strips™. A drip pad is useful to catch small volumes of bleeding.

COMPLICATIONS AND THEIR MANAGEMENT

Complications of the tongue-and-groove technique include those commonly encountered during rhinoplasty. Pertinent complications can be subdivided into intraoperative and postoperative cases. Intraoperative complications include excessive bleeding. Postoperative complications include epistaxis, infection, wound dehiscence, and asymmetry. Long-term postoperative complications include the need for revisions.

It is important to understand the implications of perioperative bleeding as well as ways of controlling excessive bleeding intraoperatively. Aside from the health risk and inconvenience of epistaxis, excessive bleeding intraoperatively can result in greater edema and postoperative ecchymosis and increased scarring. If patients consume medications known to cause bleeding or have risks factors for vitamin K deficiency, medications can be discontinued preoperatively and/or vitamin K supplementation can be administered. Basic intraoperative techniques for controlling bleeding include the use of local anesthesia containing epinephrine, gentle packing with gauze soaked in vasoconstrictive agents, tight blood pressure control, appropriate depth of general anesthesia, and prudent use of intravenous fluids. If excessive bleeding occurs, 0.3 μg/kg DDAVP (desmopressin acetate) dissolved in 50 to 75 mL of injectable saline can be infused over 30 to 45 minutes. Absolute contraindication to the use of DDAVP is the presence of coronary artery disease. As an alternative, if the patient forms clots that are not strong, a fibrinolytic disorder may be present, and infusion of aminocaproic acid may prove useful at a dose of 4 to 5 g in 250 mL of saline.[25–28]

Postoperative bleeding is controlled with similar measures. Most postoperative bleeding can be managed with adequate pain control, appropriate antiemetic agents, avoidance of nausea triggers, head elevation, gentle pressure, and vasoconstrictive nasal sprays. In cases of bleeding for more than 10 to 15 minutes despite conservative measures, DDAVP can be infused in the absence of contraindications. Note that nasal packing in the postoperative phase has never been required in the senior author's 30-year experience. Patients who respond to DDAVP intraoperatively often bleed a second time at 7 to 10 days postoperatively, thus requiring a second dose of DDAVP. If aminocaproic acid was given intraoperatively, 1 g of

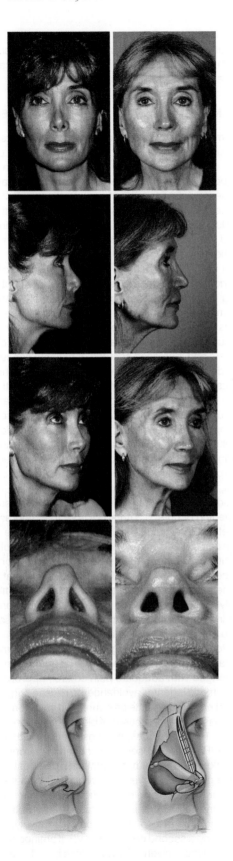

aminocaproic acid by mouth can be given every 8 hours postoperatively. Although epistaxis is common after rhinoplasty, especially if it is combined with septoplasty and turbinectomy, hematoma is exceedingly rare, given that dead space is generally obliterated.

Additional postoperative complications include infection, wound dehiscence, asymmetry, and the need for revisions. Postoperative infections occur because the surgery involves portions of the unsterile upper respiratory tract. Harbingers of late postoperative infection include intermittent bloody discharge, especially in the morning. Patients can also present with cellulitis and sinusitis. To avoid these complications, prophylactic antibiotics are routinely used. Antibiotics are especially useful when Doyle splints are in place to avoid toxic shock syndrome. Permanent sutures are used only when they are necessary. Wound dehiscence at the transcolumellar incision can occur, especially in cases of significant elongation, because the soft tissue envelope is often forced over a larger skeletal framework. Dehiscence can be reduced by avoiding tension and by using buried 6-0 poliglycaprone before aligning skin flaps at the transcolumellar incision Asymmetries can become apparent as edema subsides and the surgical framework evolves. In the longer term, revision surgery is a possibility, depending on the level of perfectionism in the patient and surgeon.[29,30]

POSTPROCEDURAL CARE

The splint and Doyle stents are typically removed after 8 days. Prophylactic first-generation cephalosporin antibiotics are given while the Doyle splints are in position. Most patients do not require taping once the splint is removed. However, if there is supratip fullness, then taping may be indicated at night for a total of 6 weeks. Steroids may be useful to prevent edema and ecchymosis. If there are no contraindications, such as acne, patients are given 10 mg of dexamethasone intraoperatively and a Medrol dose pack postoperatively. It should be emphasized to patients that soft tissue edema is still expected and can last for up to a year postoperatively. Patients are

◀───────────────────────

Fig. 5. A patient before (*left column*) and 12 years after (*right column*) elongation of a secondary short nose using the tongue-and-groove technique. The illustrations shows the soft tissue and frame alterations needed to achieve the intended goals. (*From* Guyuron B. Elongation of the short nose. In: Guyuron B, editor. Rhinoplasty. New York: Elsevier; 2012. p. 187–8; with permission.)

instructed to refrain from strenuous activity or any kind of heavy lifting for 3 weeks. Glasses are not to be worn for 5 weeks.

REHABILITATION AND RECOVERY

The aesthetic appearance of the operated nose is constantly evolving, which must be emphasized to the patient. In general, the nose should appear close to optimal a year after surgery, so revision surgery should not be considered until much later.

It is also important to emphasize that patient compliance with postoperative instructions can influence the surgical outcome significantly. Patients who smoke experience a loss of skin elasticity and thickness more quickly in the cephalic half of the nose, and they are predisposed to developing a supratip deformity secondary to sebaceous hyperplasia. Sun exposure accelerates aging and reduces skin elasticity, which can reveal minor imperfections in the nasal frame over time. Given the rigidity of the tongue-and-groove construct, the underlying framework can result in skin thinning over time.

Several flaws can become apparent in the extended recovery period for patients undergoing elongation procedures, many of which are important to rhinoplasty in general. Nasal base rigidity is one potential pitfall, especially if extended spreader grafts are sutured to the columellar strut. As previously mentioned, alar retraction is another potential pitfall that can be seen when lateral tissues are not properly advanced or excessive central lengthening is performed. Violation of nasal muscles can result in dynamic nasal imperfections with animation over time.

OUTCOMES

Fig. 5 shows a patient before and 12 years after elongation of a secondary short nose using the tongue-and-groove technique. The soft tissue and frame alterations needed to achieve the intended goals can be seen. The following maneuvers were performed: external approach, low-low osteotomy, tongue-and-groove construct, medial crura approximation, onlay tip grafting, dorsal grafting, and bilateral alar rim grafting. Video 2 highlights these maneuvers.

CLINICAL RESULTS IN THE LITERATURE

Several articles highlight iterations of techniques included in the algorithm presented in this article. Dingman and Walter[31] and Gruber[32] described composite conchal grafts for nasal lengthening. Gunter and Rohrich[33] eloquently describe caudal derotation of the lower lateral cartilages to achieve

Table 1 Case series of nasal elongation using the tongue-and-groove technique	
# Patients	27
# Patients with follow-up	23
# Previous rhinoplasties	8 were primary, 15 were secondary
# Follow-up (mo)	11–149
# Excellent results	12
# Fair results	2

Data from Guyuron B, Varghai A. Lengthening the nose with a tongue-and-groove technique. Plast Reconstr Surg 2003;111:1533–9.

lengthening. Hamra[34] describes used of single or stacked tip grafts to add length in cases of mild shortening. Several other excellent reviews are present in the literature.[35,36] However, almost all reports on the topic of nasal elongation focus on algorithms or case examples, with few discrete patient data.

In study published by our group, 27 patients underwent tongue-and-groove constructs. Twenty three were available for follow-up. Patients' ages ranged from 14 to 68 years, with an average of 31 years. Eight were primary rhinoplasties, and the remainder were secondary. The duration of follow-up ranged from 11 months to 149 months, with an average of 31 months. By the senior author's assessment, 12 patients had excellent results, 8 had good results, and 2 had fair results. Both of the patients with fair results underwent revision. Among patients requiring revision, all except for 1 occurred during the earliest stage of the senior author's experience with the tongue-and-groove technique. Significant secondary scarring was noted during these revision rhinoplasties. These results are summarized in Table 1.

SUMMARY

Three different categories of technique are available for nasal elongation. For mild anterior nasal length deficiency, we prefer a shield-type graft that does not extend over the domes unless there is projection deficiency present at the same time. In cases of moderate to severe length deficiency, the tongue-and-groove technique of nasal lengthening is a versatile technique that offers predictable and stable results on a supple nasal base. If accurate diagnosis of the specific deformity is accomplished, correction of even severe length deficiencies is possible. Lateral crural repositioning, alar rim grafting, or lateral crural strut grafting may need to be used if alar retraction is a concern.

Potential limitations of the tongue-and-groove technique include the time-intensive nature of the procedure. Alar dynamics are important considerations when planning central lengthening, and ancillary techniques need to be used to ensure that nasal elongation is achieved by the most balanced means possible.

QUESTIONS

1. How is nasal length quantified, and what are the features of a short nose?
2. How is mild anterior length deficiency corrected?
3. How is moderate to severe length deficiency corrected?
4. What are the key components of the tongue-and-groove technique?

SUPPLEMENTARY DATA

Supplementary data related to this article can be found online at http://dx.doi.org/10.1016/j.fsc. 2014.09.006.

REFERENCES

1. Janis JE, Rohrich RJ. Rhinoplasty. In: Thorne CH, Beasley RW, Aston SJ, et al, editors. Grabb and Smith's plastic surgery. 6th edition. Philadelphia: Wolters Kluwer Health/Lippincott Williams & Wilkins; 2007. p. 517–32.
2. Rohrich RJ, Hoxworth RE. Primary rhinoplasty. In: Guyuron B, Erikkson E, Persing JA, et al, editors. Plastic surgery: indications and practice. Philadelphia: Elsevier; 2009. p. 1479–508.
3. Guyuron B. Patient assessment for rhinoplasty. In: Guyuron B, editor. Rhinoplasty. New York: Elsevier; 2012. p. 27–60.
4. Guyuron B. Dynamics in rhinoplasty. Plast Reconstr Surg 2000;105(6):2259.
5. Guyuron B. Dynamics of rhinoplasty. Plast Reconstr Surg 1991;88(6):970–8.
6. Guyuron B. Dynamics of rhinoplasty. In: Guyuron B, editor. Rhinoplasty. New York: Elsevier; 2012. p. 61–97.
7. Ponsky DC, Harvey DJ, Khan SW, et al. Nose elongation: a review and description of the septal extension tongue-and-groove technique. Aesthet Surg J 2010;30(3):335–46.
8. Gruber RP. The short nose. Clin Plast Surg 1996;23: 297–313.
9. Byrd HS, Burt JD, Yazdani A, et al. Lengthening the short nose. In: Gunter JP, Rohrich RJ, Adams WP, editors. Dallas rhinoplasty: nasal surgery by the masters. 2nd edition. St Louis (MO): Quality Medical Publishing; 2007. p. 1049–62.
10. Guyuron B. Classification and operative guide to posttraumatic nasal injuries: invited personal perspective. J Craniofac Surg 2001;7(1):32–41.
11. Guyuron B, Afrooz PN. Correction of cocaine-related nasal defects. Plast Reconstr Surg 2008; 121:1015–23.
12. Zweibel SJ, Lee M, Alleyne B, et al. The incidence of vitamin, mineral, herbal, and other supplement use in facial cosmetic patients. Plast Reconstr Surg 2013;132:78–82.
13. Behin F, Behin B, Bigal ME, et al. Surgical treatment of patients with refractory migraine headaches and intranasal contact points. Cephalalgia 2005;25(6): 439–43.
14. Welge-Luessen A, Hauser R, Schmid N, et al. Endonasal surgery for contact point headaches: a 10-year longitudinal study. Laryngoscope 2003;113(12): 2151–6.
15. Guyuron B. Rhinogenic migraine headaches. In: Guyuron B, editor. Rhinoplasty. New York: Elsevier; 2012. p. 180–9, 442–7.
16. Armijo BS, Brown M, Guyuron B. Defining the ideal nasolabial angle. Plast Reconstr Surg 2012;129(3): 759–64.
17. Brown M, Guyuron B. Redefining the ideal nasolabial angle: part 2. Expert analysis. Plast Reconstr Surg 2013;132(2):221–5.
18. Guyuron B. Precision rhinoplasty: part I. The role of life-size photographs and soft-tissue cephalometric analysis. Plast Reconstr Surg 1988;81:489–99.
19. Guyuron B. Elongation of the short nose. In: Guyuron B, editor. Rhinoplasty. New York: Elsevier; 2012. p. 180–9.
20. Guyuron B. Primary rhinoplasty. In: Guyuron B, editor. Rhinoplasty. New York: Elsevier; 2012. p. 104–31.
21. Guyuron B, Jackowe D. Modified tip grafts and tip punch devices. Plast Reconstr Surg 2007;120: 2004–10.
22. Guyuron B. Alar rim deformities. Plast Reconstr Surg 2001;107(3):856–63.
23. Guyuron B, Ghavami A, Wishnek SM. Components of the short nostril. Plast Reconstr Surg 2005; 116(5):1517–23.
24. Guyuron B, Varghai A. Lengthening the nose with a tongue-and groove technique. Plast Reconstr Surg 2003;111:1533–9.
25. Guyuron B. Prevention and management of postoperative complications in rhinoplasty. In: Guyuron B, editor. Rhinoplasty. New York: Elsevier; 2012. p. 430–40.
26. Totonchi A, Eshraghi Y, Beck D, et al. Von Willebrand disease: screening, diagnosis, and management. Aesthet Surg J 2008;28(2):189–94.
27. Guyuron B, Zarandy S, Tirgan A. Von Willebrand's disease and plastic surgery. Ann Plast Surg 1994; 32(4):351–5.
28. Faber C, Larson K, Amirlak B, et al. Use of desmopressin for unremitting epistaxis following

septorhinoplasty and turbinectomy. Plast Reconstr Surg 2011;128(6):728e–32e.

29. Ponsky D, Eshraghi Y, Guyuron B. The frequency of surgical maneuvers during open rhinoplasty. Plast Reconstr Surg 2010;126(1):240–4.

30. Guyuron B. Rhinoplasty and time element. In: Guyuron B, editor. Rhinoplasty. New York: Elsevier; 2012. p. 430–9.

31. Dingman RO, Walter C. Use of composite ear grafts in correction of the short nose. Plast Reconstr Surg 1969;43:117–24.

32. Gruber RP. Surgical correction of the short nose. Aesthetic Plast Surg 2002;26(Suppl 1):S6.

33. Gunter JP, Rohrich RJ. Lengthening the aesthetically short nose. Plast Reconstr Surg 1989;83:793–800.

34. Hamra ST. Lengthening the foreshortened nose. Plast Reconstr Surg 2001;108:547–9.

35. Naficy S, Baker SR. Lengthening the short nose. Arch Otolaryngol Head Neck Surg 1998;124:809–13.

36. Toriumi DM, Patel AB, DeRosa J. Correcting the short nose in revision rhinoplasty. Facial Plast Surg Clin North Am 2006;14:343–55.

Nasal Tip Deprojection with Crural Cartilage Overlap: The M-Arch Model

Noah Benjamin Sands, MD, FRCSC[a,b],
Peter A. Adamson, MD, FRCSC[a,b],*

KEYWORDS

- Nasal tip dynamics ● Deprojection ● M-arch model ● Vertical lobule division ● Vertical arch division

KEY POINTS

- The M-arch model is a contemporary expansion of the nasal tip tripod theory, which helps to provide a conceptual framework for understanding the anatomy and dynamics of the alar cartilages.
- Shortening the M-arch, effected by vertical arch division at a carefully chosen point along the contour of the alar cartilages, can help to achieve substantial, controlled, and predictable adjustments in projection and rotation, producing refinement of the tip when indicated.
- After vertical arch division, reconstitution and overlap of the split ends of the alar cartilage maintains normal anatomy and strength, limits postoperative shifting, and allows the tip to remain stable in its optimal position.
- Depending on the distance of the vertical arch division from the tip defining point, the relative effects on deprojection, rotation, and tip refinement can be determined.
- Divisions closer to the lobule have a greater effect on narrowing the lobule, and to a lesser degree on rotation, whereas the reverse principal applies when divisions are placed further from the tip.

INTRODUCTION

The nasal tip is widely appreciated by rhinoplasty surgeons as the most conceptually and technically challenging aspect of the nose to master. The vast number of tip-altering techniques used to modify and establish the 3 principal parameters of nasal aesthetics—length, projection, and rotation—is a testament to the complexity and level of difficulty involved in surgically controlling the lower third of the nose. As is frequently the case when applying challenging and intricate surgical principles in practice, simplification is often a reliable path to understanding. It is for this reason that rudimentary concepts tend to withstand the test of time, amid a myriad of more complicated paradigms. One seemingly eternal simplification of tip dynamics, Jack R. Anderson's nasal tip tripod concept (1969),[1] has greatly advanced the universal understanding of the tip among rhinoplasty surgeons and has facilitated the development of various techniques. This tripod concept defines the

The authors have no conflicts of interest or disclosures.
This material has never been published and is not currently under evaluation in any other peer-reviewed publication.
[a] Division of Facial Plastic and Reconstructive Surgery, Department of Otolaryngology – Head and Neck Surgery, University of Toronto, Toronto General Hospital, R. Fraser Elliott Building, 190 Elizabeth Street, Room 3S – 438, Toronto, Ontario M5G 2C4, Canada; [b] Adamson Associates Cosmetic Facial Surgery, 150 Bloor Street West, M110, Toronto, Ontario M5S 2X9, Canada
* Corresponding author.
E-mail address: paa@dradamson.com

conjoined medial crura (MC) as the central leg of a tripod and the lower lateral crura (LC) as the 2 side legs. The position of the tip-defining point (TDP) can be manipulated by altering the length(s) of these legs (**Fig. 1**). Shortening the legs decreases projection (retrodisplacement) and, depending on the integrated degree of shortening of the MC and LC, there will be a variable effect on rotation and, subsequently, on nasal length.

The M-arch model, first described by the senior author in 2006,[2] expands on the concept of the nasal tip tripod by conceptualizing the tip as continuous paired arches. This model is more accurate, both anatomically and dynamically, when considering the actual architecture of the tip, and provides for a more detailed and utilitarian approach to the application of surgical techniques. The essence of the model is that these paired arches have a specific length. Furthermore, each of the components of the M-arch—the MC, intermediate crura (IC), and LC—has a length. These component lengths, and their combined overall length, establish tip projection and rotation, and indirectly nasal length. Shortening the length of the M-arch, implemented by vertical division at a carefully chosen point along its contour, can help to achieve substantial, controlled, and predictable adjustments in projection and rotation, while also producing refinement of the tip when indicated. The senior author has gradually evolved toward the application of crural cartilage overlap (overlay) techniques, in lieu of division or excision, with or without end-to-end reconstitution of the cartilage, as was typically performed in the past. Overlap of the alar cartilage helps to strengthen and spatially fixate the alar cartilages, and ultimately the tip complex, producing more reliable positioning of the TDP. In cases where the arch length needs to be increased, a variety of cartilage grafts and steal techniques are applied to increase the relative lengths of the M-arch components. Herein, we

have addressed the use of crural overlay techniques to decrease the length of the arch, thereby achieving our desired projection, rotation, nasal length, and lobule definition. The M-arch model does not directly address changes in tip projection and rotation effected by maneuvers that weaken the support structures of the tip, such as transfixion incision or weakening of ligaments in the intercrural or scroll regions or excision of premaxillary spine. However, if these maneuvers or others are performed, their effects can be integrated easily into the M-arch model by invoking how they individually affect the length of the specific M-arch components.

NASAL TIP ANATOMY AND DEFINITIONS

The nasal tip is composed of the conjoined MC, IC, and diverging lower LC (**Fig. 2**). The TDPs, which are highlighted by an external light reflex, are formed by the apices, or most anterior projections, of the domal arches, which have varying degrees of acuity related to the underlying shape and angulation of the alar cartilages.

The nasal lobule includes the soft tissue anterior to the nostril apex, caudal to the supratip break of the dorsum, and anterior to the lateral alar side walls. The lobule can be subdivided into the supratip, infratip, and paired lateral supratips, each of which neighbors the TDPs. The nasal base includes the infratip lobule, columella, alar side walls, and nasal sill.

Beyond the cartilages, the thickness or thinness of the skin–soft tissue envelope (S-STE) has a significant impact on the degree of tip definition. Thin skin reveals the details of cartilage anatomy, whereas thick skin blunts the appearance of well-defined domes, both for the better or worse.

The cephalic border of the nasal tip is the transition into the scroll region, or junction of the LC with the caudal upper lateral cartilage, via fibrous attachments. The caudal edge of the tip consists of the soft tissue triangles of the alar rims, which extend below the caudal margin of the alar cartilages. The lateral edge of the tip is the transition into the alar–facial groove and bony pyriform fossa. With respect to additional attachments, the MC cartilages are fixed onto the posterior septal angle, and extend anteriorly to the apex of the nostrils, which correspond to the medial crural angle (junction of the MC and IC). The medial crural angle follows a gentle curvature to transition seamlessly with the IC, which is defined as the segment of the tip cartilage that extends from the medial crural angle to the TDP. The lateral crus extends from the TDP to the hinge area, or junction of the LC with the pyriform fossa (see **Fig. 2**). Sesamoid cartilage

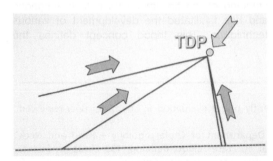

Fig. 1. Jack R. Anderson's tripod concept. The position of the tip-defining point (TDP) can be altered by changing the relative lengths of the medial and lower lateral crura. These changes alter thrusting forces and ultimately determine the position of the tip.

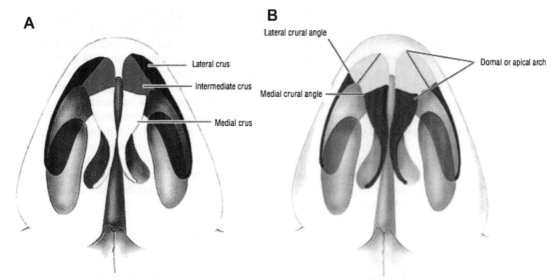

Fig. 2. Anatomy of the M-arch model. (*A*) The M-arch consists of the conjoined medial crura and intermediate crura (IC) and the bilateral lower lateral crura (LC). (*B*) The domal arch is formed unilaterally by the IC, anterior aspect of the LC, and external and internal soft tissue triangles. The conjoined domal arches constitute the lobular arch. (*From* Funk E, Chauhan N, Adamson PA. Refining vertical lobule division in open septorhinoplasty. Arch Facial Plast Surg 2009;11(2):120–5; with permission.)

may be present at this transition point. This area is also called the foot of the LC, analogous to the foot of the MC, where the MC embraces the posterior septal angle.

Although neighboring anatomic structures transmit their intrinsic forces to the tip by way of ligamentous and fascial attachments, influencing its overall appearance, the underlying structure of the alar cartilages constitutes the foundation and primary determinant of nasal tip anatomy and its dynamics. Its construct can be altered by surgical refinements guided by the tripod concept and the M-arch model. The M-arch anatomy can be best described as a pair of adjoining arches in much the same way as the "golden arches" of the McDonald's Restaurant Corporation (Oak Brook, IL). This symbol is widely recognized and thus serves as a useful tool to represent both the anatomic construct of the alar cartilages as well as the impact of surgical modifications. An important feature of the M-arch is that the lateral legs of the alar cartilages are not in the same horizontal plane as the medial legs, but rather oriented in a posterosuperior position. As described in the senior author's original article, the golden arches facing a headwind would best illustrate the anatomic configuration of these cartilages.[2]

From an anatomic perspective, one of the major advantages of the M-arch model, with respect to the more classic tripod concept, includes its consideration of the tip as a continuous arch, as

opposed to a 3 straight-legged structure. It also recognizes the importance of the medial, intermediate, and lateral crural arches in continuity, instead of the MC and LC being attached at a hinge. The M-arch model defines yet another arch, the domal arch. This is essentially an arch within an arch, and consists of the intermediate crus (ie, the IC) and anterior component of the LC. The M-arch concept's inclusion of the intermediate crus, and subsequently its consideration of how alterations in the arch can affect lobule definition, is an additional advantage. The tripod concept predates the labeling of the intermediate crus and simply does not address the lobule.

NASAL TIP DYNAMICS

In essence, the goal of rhinoplasty is to alter the architecture of the bony and cartilaginous structure of the nose to create an underlying foundation for the S-STE to redrape. The resultant aesthetic of the nose is largely contingent on appropriately addressing the 3 fundamental parameters—length, projection, and rotation—which are determined by the position of the TDPs, and the balance of these parameters with tip refinement, as well as the construct of the nasal dorsum and nasal base.

The tip receives its structural support from a multitude of sources, none greater than the size, shape, strength, and resiliency of the alar cartilages themselves.[3] The curvature of the conjoined medial and LC, which include the IC, creates an inborn tension in the structure, somewhat like a "sprung horseshoe."[2] The LC provides anterior tension to the tip, thrusting the complex anteriorly and inferiorly. This vector is counteracted and stabilized by the anterior and superior thrusting force of the MC. The ultimate position of the TDP is primarily determined by the resultant vector of these 2 forces, modified by the intrinsic strength of the cartilage (**Fig. 3**). Additional sources of support include the attachment of the feet of the MC with the posterior septal angle, the scroll region, the hinge area of the LC, and the interdomal ligaments.

With respect to tip dynamics, the M-arch model is more elaborate than the tripod theory in describing the impact of surgical adjustments on the major parameters of the tip. The M-arch model also lends itself to more comprehensive technical descriptions of methods that alter arch length, including lengthening procedures. These methods influence the 3 major aesthetic parameters to a variable degree, depending on the amount of M-arch alteration, and the distance and direction from the TDPs. It is important for the rhinoplasty surgeon to recognize the capacity of each of these maneuvers, irrespective of the degree of simplicity or complexity, to impact all of the major parameters of the tip, and not simply projection. That

said, the capacity to bring about changes in projection, and in particular deprojection of the tip in patients with marked overprojection, is a unifying feature of the majority of these M-arch–altering techniques. Although a slightly overprojected nose can frequently be addressed by interrupting the support mechanisms itemized herein, M-arch shortening is especially valuable to address the highly overprojected tip that demands a greater degree of deprojection, or when multiple parameters require alteration in unison, including the need for considerable lobular refinement. M-arch shortening can impart powerful changes to these parameters.

TRIPOD CONCEPT AND TIP DEPROJECTION

The purpose of the Tripod concept is to allow one to conceptualize maneuvers that first alter tip projection, secondarily impact tip rotation, and ultimately establish nasal length. The tripod concept did not originally consider the effect of lengthening the crural legs to add projection. Instead, it described the aesthetic result of incising or shortening, without reconstitution, either the MC or LC at their footplate attachments to the posterior septal angle and hinge area, respectively. Shortening both components could also be performed in conjunction. Incising the lateral crus near the hinge area decreases the thrusting force of this leg of the tripod, thereby decreasing projection and effecting some rotation. Greater amounts of deprojection and rotation can be achieved by excision of a segment of the lateral crural feet (rim strip technique, first described by Webster and Smith[4]). These rotational maneuvers also shorten the length of the nose.

Incising or shortening the MC at their base can achieve deprojection and counter-rotation of the tip, which ultimately increases nasal length. The posterior septal angle, at its junction with the footplates, can be excised to obtain minimal changes in these parameters, whereas a more substantial alteration in tip position can be effected by excising a portion of the medial crus itself at the level of the feet. The overall effect on the position of the TDPs is determined by the sum and relative amount of shortening imparted on the MC, IC, and LC. In general, small amounts of length reduction in any aspect of the tripod, in the order of 1 to 3 mm, can achieve measurable changes in tip parameters, with changes in projection being paramount.[5] Each of these techniques avoids a division in the central portion of the M-arch, and instead creates a skeletal void at one (or both) of the terminal ends to permit tip deprojection and altered rotation. However, the void created could

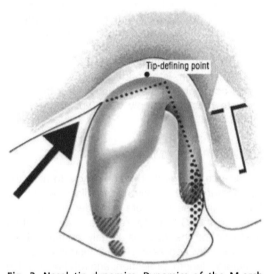

Fig. 3. Nasal tip dynamics. Dynamics of the M-arch showing the thrusting forces (*arrows*) of the medial crura and lateral crura that define the position of the tip-defining point. This dimension, in turn, defines projection, rotation and (indirectly) length. (*From* Funk E, Chauhan N, Adamson PA. Refining vertical lobule division in open septorhinoplasty. Arch Facial Plast Surg 2009;11(2):120–5; with permission.)

lead to unpredictable postoperative migration of the tip and a variable degree of deprojection that is determined largely by various tip suspensory forces, instead of by the judgment and skill of the surgeon.

M-ARCH MODEL: DEPROJECTION WITH VERTICAL ARCH DIVISION AND CRURAL OVERLAP

The M-arch model is an expansion of the tripod concept both in terms of its anatomic realism and description of tip dynamics. Because the model is more contemporary and elaborate compared with the tripod concept, so are the surgical techniques that have been described to alter its parameters—particularly projection. These techniques include interruptions, referred to as vertical arch divisions, along any portion of the M-arch, and not just incisions or trimmings of cartilage at the terminal segments. These divisions allow for more powerful and predictable maneuvering of the tip. After division, the ends of the alar cartilage can be left free floating, reapproximated end-to-end after removal of a segment, or fixated in an overlapped orientation. The senior author has migrated exclusively toward the latter procedure over the spectrum of his career.

A vertical division is an incision in the M-arch perpendicular to the long axis of the arch. This is in contradistinction to a horizontal division, parallel to the long axis of the arch. The most classic example of a horizontal division is the horizontal cephalic trim of the alar cartilages used to refine the lobule and/or achieve minimal rotation. Examples of commonly employed vertical divisions include cartilaginous incisions placed in the hinge area (hinge incision/excision), mid portion of the LC (lateral crural flap or overlay), within the lobular arch itself (vertical lobule division [VLD] or intermediate crural overlay), within the mid portion of the MC (medial crural overlay) or at the base of the MC (medial crural incision/excision; **Fig. 4**).

The lateral crural flap technique, originally described by Webster and Smith,[4] was designed as a closed approach to achieve substantial tip rotation and deprojection, while limiting the potential for postoperative tip migration into a spatial void. The division and cartilage trim is imparted on the lateral crus cephalic to its divergence from the alar rim, preserving a segment of cartilage in continuity with the hinge area, which serves as a crutch for the free edge. Like the rim strip technique, the free edge of the lateral crus is left unfixed and mobile, which can result in

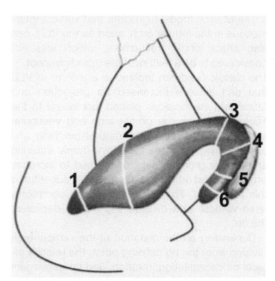

Fig. 4. Vertical arch division. The various locations of more common M-arch divisions. (1) Lateral crural hinge area. (2) Mid portion of the lateral crus (lateral crural overlay). (3) Vertical lobule division (VLD; Goldman division). (4) VLD (intermediate crural overlay). (5) Medial crura (medial crural overlay). (6) Medial crural foot. (*From* Funk E, Chauhan N, Adamson PA. Refining vertical lobule division in open septorhinoplasty. Arch Facial Plast Surg 2009;11(2):120–5; with permission.)

movement, telescoping, and asymmetry in the postoperative setting. The free edge is also capable of flaring outward, causing external fullness postoperatively, or prolapsing into the nasal vestibule, contributing to functional obstruction. It is the concern over such complications that has compelled the senior author to overlap (overlay) the divided ends of the M-arch, and secure them by suturing, as Kridel and Konior[6] advised in their description of the lateral crural overlay technique to address the overprojected, ptotic tip. It is also a modification of VLD with overlay the senior author has been using through most of his career.[7] The senior author uses this overlay approach, without resection of cartilage, invariably and irrespective of location along the M-arch. Avoiding resection, and employing reconstitution of the split ends in this overlapping manner, helps to preserve crural cartilage volume and strength, maintains "normal" alar cartilage anatomy, limits postoperative shifting secondary to contraction and fibrosis, and ultimately allows the tip to remain stable in its optimal positioning. With the open rhinoplasty approach, precise suturing is performed with relative ease under direct vision and generally constitutes the modern standard when applying vertical arch divisions.

The M-arch model highlights that vertical interruptions in the lobular arch, such as the VLD, can also affect lobular refinement, which was not considered to be a feature of the tripod concept.[5,7] The classic Goldman technique is a form of VLD that can achieve increased tip projection and refinement via incisions placed just lateral to the TDP but through the domal arch and vestibular skin.[8] Owing to risks of unnatural pinching and alar notching, more conservative domal suturing and lobular grafting techniques used to increase projection and refinement have largely substituted this technique. The remainder of the commonly used vertical arch division techniques deproject the tip.

Depending on the distance of the vertical arch division from the tip defining point, the relative effects on deprojection, rotation, and tip refinement can be determined (**Fig. 5** and case presentations in **Figs. 6–8**). Divisions closer to the lobule have a greater effect on narrowing the lobule, and to a lesser degree on rotation, whereas the reverse principal applies when divisions are placed further from the tip and closer to the feet.

VLD with cartilage overlap (intermediate crural overlay), performed by the senior author, is typically placed within the IC to impart changes in tip projection and refinement, while minimally affecting rotation. This technique has additional capabilities, such as correcting tip asymmetries, reducing the hanging infratip lobule, refining the broad domal arch, and improving the columellar–lobular relationship. Depending on the exact placement of the VLD, different objectives can be met. If placed near the angle of the MC and IC, just medial to the TDPs at the medial crural angle, vertical shortening of the lobule with deprojection is achieved along with some refinement. When positioned closer to the tip defining points, VLD effects primarily lobular shortening and narrowing, with less of an influence on projection (see **Fig. 5; Fig. 9**). This variable effect of VLD by location is related to the orientation of the alar cartilages in the coronal plane of face, where both horizontal and vertical components exist. Projection is effected more by changes in the vertical vector (VLD medial to the TDP), whereas lobular refinement is primarily achieved by shortening the horizontal component of the arch or narrowing the breadth of the lobule by placing the VLD directly at the TDP. Both of these techniques are globally considered "VLDs."

One particularly difficult problem to address in rhinoplasty is asymmetry of the tip lobule. The

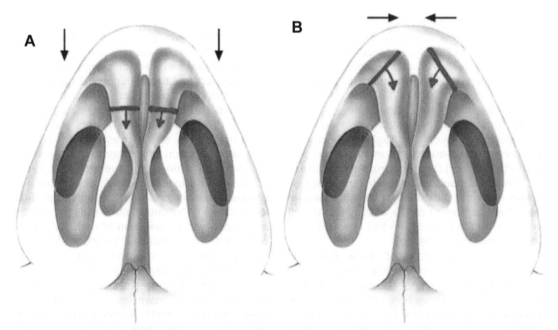

Fig. 5. Effects of vertical lobule division (VLD) with intermediate crural overlay (ICO) placed within the domal arch. (*A*) The overlap is performed in the domal arch, at the poorly defined junction between the medial crura (MC) and intermediate crura (IC; medial crural angle). In this region, the M-arch has a significant vertical component, allowing the VLD to primarily deproject and counter-rotate the tip. (*B*) The overlap is performed near the tip-defining point, where there is a significant horizontal component to the M-arch, resulting primarily in lobular narrowing of a broad lobule. (*From* Funk E, Chauhan N, Adamson PA. Refining vertical lobule division in open septorhinoplasty. Arch Facial Plast Surg 2009;11(2):120–5; with permission.)

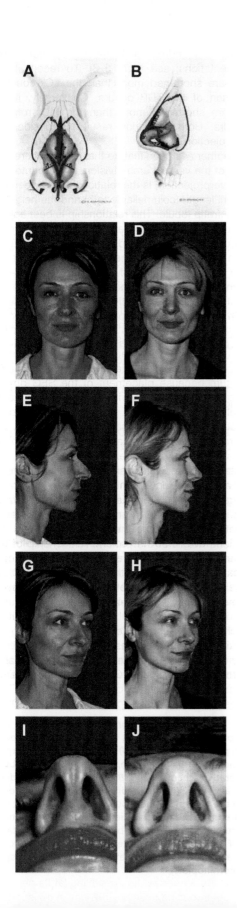

VLD is also a useful tool in the management of tip asymmetries because it addresses each dome individually and to a variable degree. Unilateral arch shortening can help to address knuckling or redundancy on 1 side and unilateral narrowing can be carried out for a splayed dome that is out of proportion to the other, among other possible modifications. Overlap and strengthening of the dome(s) can also help to prevent repeated knuckling and asymmetries.

Overlap and stabilization of the crura with sutures is particularly important in the vicinity of the domal arch to help reliably lock the tip in its new position, while preventing postoperative irregularities, knuckling, and asymmetries. Even when the arch division is more remote from the domal arch, overlap and suturing the cut ends together helps to ensure the new nasal tip position.

The senior author utilizes vertical arch divisions with overlap, placed closer to either the MC (medial crural overlay) or LC (lateral crural overlay) feet (**Fig. 10**) to more dramatically alter projection and rotation without impacting lobular refinement. The anticipated effects of these techniques on the major aesthetic parameters of the nose has already been discussed by way of individual or combined leg shortening of the nasal tripod. Any division and overlap lateral to the TDP results in deprojection, rotation, and shortening of the nose; likewise, any division medial to the TDP deprojects, counter-rotates, and elongates the nose. The degree of change in each of these parameters is contingent on the distance from the TDP that the division is made and the amount of overlap applied to the medial and lateral ends. The ability to tailor these alterations bestows on the surgeon considerable control over the resultant position of the tip.

These techniques can be applied alone or in combination, and with or without VLD for lobular

Fig. 6. Illustrations (*A, B*) and preoperative photographs (*C, E, G, I*) and postoperative photographs (*D, F, H, J*) of a patient with a markedly overprojected and counter-rotated nose. Operative schematics (*A, B*) illustrating medial crural shortening and lateral crural overlay to decrease the length of the M-arch. This helps to obtain selective deprojection and rotation with shortening of the nose. A columellar strut graft was placed to maintain projection and interdomal sutures were applied for minor lobule refinement and stability. Frontal (*C, D*), right lateral (*E, F*), right oblique (*G, H*), and basal (*I, J*) views before and 1 year after open septorhinoplasty.

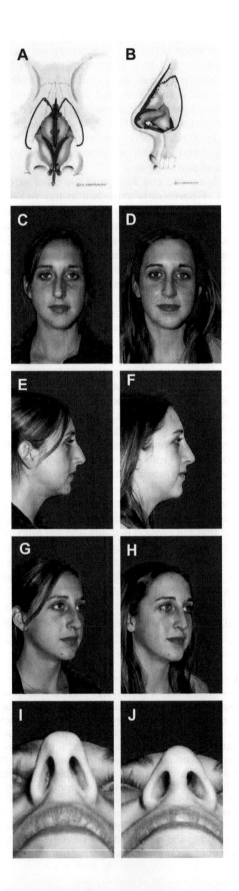

refinement and/or additional deprojection (case presentations; see **Figs. 6–8**). To recap, if the MC are shortened more than the LC, counter-rotation of the TDP occurs. Conversely, if the LC are shortened more than the MC, rotation occurs. Both scenarios result in considerable deprojection.

Another aesthetic feature that can be altered by way of the vertical arch division, in the context of tip overprojection, is the relationship between the nostril length (columellar length) and the height of the infratip lobule. This relationship is best appreciated on basal view, and the respective ratio should be 2:1 (Powell and Humphries[9]). In patients with an overly long columella, medial crural overlay can shorten the length of the central leg of the M-arch, thus shortening the length of the MC and nostrils while deprojecting the tip. In patients with an excessive infratip lobule, VLD followed by crural overlay medial to the TDP but within the lobular arch shortens the lobule. Both maneuvers deproject the tip and achieve balance between these anatomic proportions. VLD within the intermediate crus can also be applied to diminish a hanging infratip lobule.

PROCEDURAL STEPS: DEPROJECTION WITH VERTICAL ARCH DIVISION

Detailed preoperative assessment and planning, as always, is fundamental in achieving optimal surgical results. Considerations when analyzing the patient physically, and through preoperative photography, include the aesthetic goals of the patient, height of the patient, relationship of the nose to other projections of the face (forehead, maxilla, and chin), aesthetic nasal parameters, and skin thickness. Potential causes of over-projection should be elucidated; in particular, an excessive M-arch, but other contributors such as tip tension (excessive quadrangular cartilage), elongated nasal spine, and maxillary prominence should be evaluated. If the M-arch is found to be excessive in length, preoperative

Fig. 7. Schematic procedural illustrations (*A, B*) and preoperative photographs (*C, E, G, I*) and postoperative photographs (*D, F, H, J*) of a patient with overprojection, normal rotation, and a broad lobule. Operative schematics (*A, B*) illustrating intermediate crural overlay (ICO) to shorten the M-arch, deproject the tip, and refine the lobule. A columellar strut was placed to maintain projection, and interdomal sutures were placed for further lobule refinement and stability. Frontal (*C, D*), right lateral (*E, F*), right oblique (*G, H*), and basal (*I, J*) views before and 1 year after open septorhinoplasty.

contemplation of a vertical arch division should take place.

To help guide the surgeon in planning for the appropriate placement of the vertical arch division, the surgeon should consider the requirement for adjustments in projection, rotation, nasal length, and tip refinement as well as adjunctive features such as a hanging columella, redundant infratip lobule, and excessively long nostrils, each of which can be addressed via cartilage overlay. This evaluation process should again take place at the time of surgery.

An open rhinoplasty approach is used to expose the cartilaginous anatomy of the tip. Accurate assessment of the alar cartilages is important to select the appropriate maneuver for deprojection. Although a closed approach is possible to achieve virtually all of the vertical arch division techniques, more complex tip deformities generally call for the application of more complex and multiple maneuvers. In such settings the open approach is very helpful, because cartilage delivery through the endonasal approach can create distortion and challenge proper arch reconstitution.

Any necessary septal work should be accomplished before addressing the tip. Soft tissue situated between the intermediate and MC is removed as the alar cartilages are divided in the midline to expose the septum. Once the septal work is completed and mucoperichondrial flaps are reapproximated, trimming of the cephalic border of the LC is completed before performing vertical arch division. Release of a potential tension tip may obviate the need for additional deprojection and should also be addressed first.

Basal support is provided by a columellar strut graft, which is frequently placed and secured between the MC using mattress polyglactin sutures before vertical arch division. This helps to secure tip positioning, stabilizes the tip complex, and prevents excessive deprojection. In other cases, a tongue-in-groove technique, fixing the MC in a

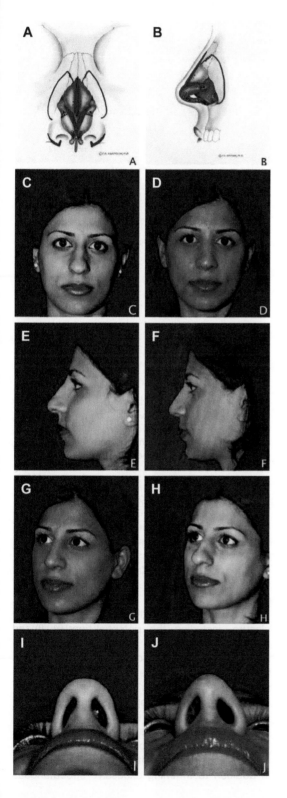

Fig. 8. Schematic procedural illustrations (*A, B*) and preoperative photographs (*C, E, G, I*) and postoperative photographs (*D, F, H, J*) of a patient with slight overprojection, normal rotation, and a markedly bulbous lobule. Operative schematics (*A, B*) illustrating shortening of a long M-arch with intermediate crural overlay (ICO) for deprojection and lobule refinement. Further deprojection and rotation was achieved with lateral crural overlay (LCO). Frontal (*C, D*), left lateral (*E, F*), left oblique (*G, H*), and basal (*I, J*) views before and 1 year after open septorhinoplasty.

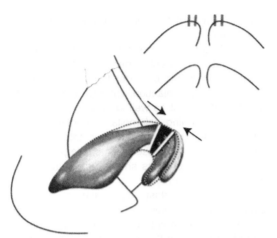

Fig. 9. Vertical lobule division (VLD) to narrow the lobule. The VLD is placed near the TDP, where there is a considerable horizontal component to the M-arch. This maneuver predominantly narrows the lobule, with less of an effect on tip deprojection. (*From* Adamson PA, Litner JA, Dahiya R. The M-Arch model: a new concept of nasal tip dynamics. Arch Facial Plast Surg 2006;8(1):16–25; with permission.)

more cephalic and either anterior or posterior position on the caudal septum, can increase or decrease the relative MC length.

Before implementing a VLD for lobule definition, consideration should be given to conservative maneuvers such as scoring, domal suturing, and tip grafting, which are frequently sufficient for tip refinement.

Before 1987, an excisional technique was used in which a portion of the M-arch was resected to alter tip position and refinement. The edges were then reapproximated and sutured end to end, without overlap. It was felt that this technique provided adequate stability to the tip; however, better techniques were constantly sought after to further prevent postoperative irregularities.[2,5,7]

After 1987, the present technique was utilized (see **Figs. 11** and **12**). This technique includes wide undermining of the vestibular skin from the alar cartilage for its preservation in the area of the anticipated division. Vertical division is then carried out at the desired site along the M-arch, preserving the vestibular skin to prevent scar contracture. Excision of a segment of cartilage is occasionally indicated, particularly in cases of tip asymmetry, including knuckling and redundancies causing excessive breadth within the domal arch. The crural ends are then realigned and overlapped 3 to 7 mm to achieve the desired changes in tip parameters. For the best possible camouflage, the

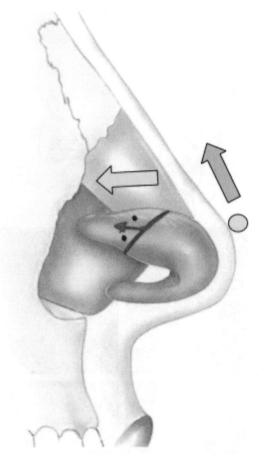

Fig. 10. Lateral crural overlay (LCO) technique of vertical arch division. The vertical division is placed within the mid portion of the lower lateral cartilage and the M-arch overlap imparts rotation and deprojection (*arrows*) of the tip-defining point (*circle*).

lateral end is advanced over the medial end after VLD and medial crural overlay, whereas the medial end is advanced over the lateral end after lateral crural overlay. The ends are then secured with 6-0 nylon horizontal mattress sutures, without inclusion of the vestibular skin. If placed within the IC, the knots are left within the interdomal space.

Final refinements in the tip are made before closure, including the potential application of lateral crural strut grafts to provide strength and symmetry, or address concavity/convexity along the alar sidewalls. These grafts are secured with mattress 4-0 polyglactin sutures placed through both ends of the overlapped cartilage, if a lateral crural overlay has already been performed, through the strut and the vestibular skin, with the knot placed in the vestibule. Finer refinements in the tip can be made with scoring and suturing, in addition to trimming excessive subcutaneous

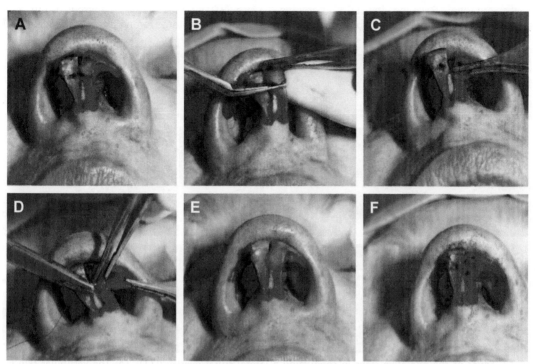

Fig. 11. Series of the operative steps in conducting an intermediate crural overlay (ICO). (*A*) The excessive M-arch is marked at the desired site of the vertical division. This corresponds with the junction of the intermediate and medial crura, medial to the tip defining point. The vestibular skin near the lobule has already been undermined. (*B*) Sharp tissue scissors shown cutting through the medial crura–intermediate crura junction on the left. (*C*) The free ends of the cartilage are overlapped to achieve the desired amount of deprojection. (*D*) Overlapped ends are fixed and stabilized with mattress sutures. (*E*) Basal view before the intermediate crural overlay. (*F*) Basal view after intermediate crural overlay performed on the left side only. (*From* Funk E, Chauhan N, Adamson PA. Refining vertical lobule division in open septorhinoplasty. Arch Facial Plast Surg 2009;11(2):120–5; with permission.)

fat before redrapage of the S-STE and finally closure.

POTENTIAL PITFALLS

The S-STE has a considerable role to play in the aesthetic outcome of any rhinoplasty. One factor the surgeon must consider when employing vertical arch divisions in thin-skinned patients, particularly within the domal arch (VLD), is the potential for postoperative contour irregularities. The senior author believes that when this concern exists, it is ideal to perform a VLD medial to the TDPs, rather than within the TDPs themselves. The overlap is subsequently camouflaged in the infratip region and rarely causes problems. If additional concealment is needed, soft tissue camouflage grafts can be applied over the VLD. In thick-skinned patients, the surgeon must recognize that even with more aggressive refinement maneuvers such as the VLD, optimal definition within the lobule may be

difficult to achieve without adjunctive measures such as structural tip grafting.

Despite the versatility of vertical arch divisions, a large cohort of surgeons has been reluctant to utilize these techniques owing to concern over postoperative irregularities. Healing of the vertically incised alar cartilage can be unpredictable owing to scarring and contracture, particularly when the ends are not secured and strengthened with overlap, as was done frequently in the past. This approach likely stigmatized vertical arch division. It should be emphasized that division and overlap provide additional strength and stability to the tip complex relative to the starting point. One study by the senior author demonstrated a 2.4% incidence of postoperative tip abnormalities using this technique.[7]

Vertical arch division could result in excessive deprojection, especially after the reduction of additional sources of tip support. Various procedures can help to "buy back" projection in such cases, such as columellar strut placement, tip grafting, or the lateral crural steal technique.[7]

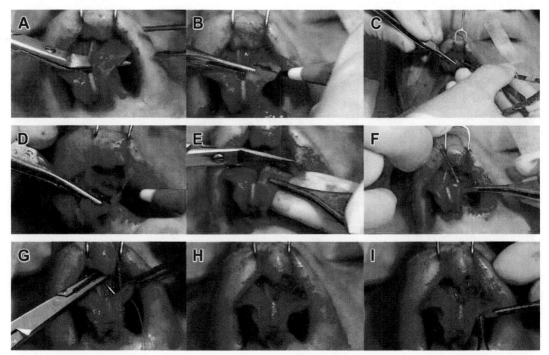

Fig. 12. Series of the operative steps in conducting a lateral crural overlay (LCO). (*A*) The vestibular skin has already been separated from the lower lateral crus (LC). (*B*) The planned incision site is marked on the LC. (*C, D*) Calipers are used to measure and mark the extent of cartilage overlay. (*E*) The LC is incised with Converse scissors. (*F*) Keith needle fixation of cartilage overlay. The vestibular skin is pulled caudally, away from the needle. (*G*) 4-0 polyglactin horizontal mattress suture fixation of the overlay. Two sutures are placed and both knots are positioned on the vestibular surface. (*H*) After LCO of the left alar cartilage, note deprojection and flattening of the LC owing to M-arch shortening. Rotation has also been affected, but is not well demonstrated here. (*I*) Note the mobility of the vestibular skin to allow marginal incision closure without creating alar retraction.

SUMMARY

Vertical arch division has been a mainstay of tip surgery for many years, and although it has been subject to multiple trends and modifications, its applications are ever expanding. It provides a particularly powerful tool for deprojection of the overprojected tip, while modifying other aesthetic parameters in a controlled, predictable fashion when the crural cartilage is preserved and overlapped, maintaining strength of the M-arch. Cartilage overlay techniques are especially apropos with respect to the central theme of modern rhinoplasty, which aims to preserve and restore normal anatomy while establishing strong support for the nasal framework that will remain over the lifespan of our patients.

REFERENCES

1. Anderson J. The dynamics of rhinoplasty. In: Bustamant G, editor. Proceedings of the Ninth International Congress of Otorhinolaryngology. Mexico City (Mexico): 1969.

2. Adamson PA, Litner JA, Dahiya R. The M-Arch model: a new concept of nasal tip dynamics. Arch Facial Plast Surg 2006;8(1):16–25.

3. Vuyk HD, Oakenfull C, Plaat RE. A quantitative appraisal of change in nasal tip projection after open rhinoplasty. Rhinology 1997;35(3):124–8.

4. Webster RC, Smith RC. Lateral crural retrodisplacement for superior rotation of the tip in rhinoplasty. Aesthetic Plast Surg 1979;3(1):65–78.

5. Funk E, Chauhan N, Adamson PA. Refining vertical lobule division in open septorhinoplasty. Arch Facial Plast Surg 2009;11(2):120–5.

6. Kridel RW, Konior RJ. Controlled nasal tip rotation via the lateral crural overlay technique. Arch Otolaryngol Head Neck Surg 1991;117(4):411–5.

7. Adamson PA, McGraw-Wall BL, Morrow TA, et al. Vertical dome division in open rhinoplasty. An update on indications, techniques, and results. Arch Otolaryngol Head Neck Surg 1994;120(4):373–80.

8. Goldman I. The importance of the mesial crura in nasal-tip reconstruction. AMA Arch Otolaryngol 1957;65(2):143–7.

9. Powell N, Humphreys B. Proportions of the aesthetic face. New York: Thieme-Stratton Inc; 1988. p. 28–30.

Index

Note: Page numbers of article titles are in **boldface** type.

Moving?

Make sure your subscription moves with you!

To notify us of your new address, find your **Clinics Account Number** (located on your mailing label above your name), and contact customer service at:

Email: journalscustomerservice-usa@elsevier.com

800-654-2452 (subscribers in the U.S. & Canada)
314-447-8871 (subscribers outside of the U.S. & Canada)

Fax number: 314-447-8029

Elsevier Health Sciences Division
Subscription Customer Service
3251 Riverport Lane
Maryland Heights, MO 63043

*To ensure uninterrupted delivery of your subscription, please notify us at least 4 weeks in advance of move.

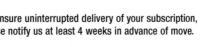

Printed and bound by CPI Group (UK) Ltd, Croydon, CR0 4YY

03/10/2024

01040374-0004